To Bob Lewis —

To the End of AIDS 2020

Bill Valenti

10·18·17

To my media colleagues —

The medium is the message

With my thanks —

AIDS: A MATTER OF URGENCY
A Doctor's Memoir

William M. Valenti, M.D.

Wm M Valenti MD

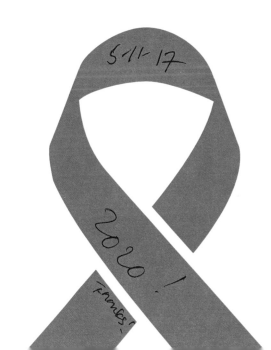

5-11-17

2020!

Thanks!

AIDS:
A MATTER
OF URGENCY

A Doctor's Memoir

William M. Valenti, M.D.
Foreword by Steven F. Scheibel, M.D.

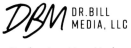 DR. BILL
MEDIA, LLC

Rochester, New York

ORDERING INFORMATION

Quantity sales. Special discounts are available on quantity purchases. For details, contact the publisher, DrBillMedia, LLC, at www.drbillvalenti.com.

Published in the United States by

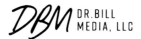 DR. BILL
MEDIA, LLC

DrBillMedia, LLC, Rochester, New York USA

ISBN 978-0-9984383-0-6 (softbound)

Printed in the United States at Mercury Print Productions on acid-free paper.
First Printing, 2017

COVER ART BY	PHOTOGRAPHY BY	BOOK DESIGN BY	EDITOR
Michael Chiazza	Matt Wittmeyer	Archer Communications	Virginia Keck

DISCLAIMER

Events described in this memoir are based on my recollections of real-life experiences. A few characters in the book are fictitious, but most are not. The real people identified, or their legal representatives, have granted me permission to use their actual names, situations, and photographs to tell this story. And to them, I am most grateful.

AUTHOR'S NOTES

This book is a compilation of patient stories and my personal memories of the early era of the AIDS epidemic, starting with the first patients in 1981. This narrative is intended to represent the mood of the 1980s, when AIDS first appeared on the scene.

I did not keep a journal. Instead, these stories are loosely compiled chronologically and describe events that are seared into my brain, many still as vivid as when they occurred. To ensure accuracy and to fill in the blanks, I referred to letters, many media interviews, and discussions with the key people involved.

There are many stories that are not included here, simply due to space constraints. Each of my patients, their families, survivors, friends, and others involved in the effort has compelling stories to tell.

The events described here and the stories still to be written have taken us from a fatal illness to talk of eliminating HIV, not only in New York State and in the United States, but around the world.

I have seen two major diseases eliminated in my lifetime: polio and smallpox. I hope AIDS will be the third.

"WHAT'S PAST IS PROLOGUE."

—*William Shakespeare*, The Tempest

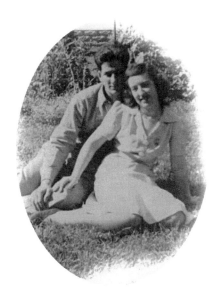

▸ Alphonse and Rose Valenti, around 1944.

DEDICATION

To my mother and father, Rose and Alphonse Valenti, who taught me the importance of hard work, perseverance, and doing good things for others.

And to my patients who taught me how to apply my parents' values for the greater good.

FOREWORD

We thought out-of-the-box and like the water streaming down the side of a mountain, the stream splits around obstacles and then reunites all its energy into the ocean for the ultimate goal of a cure for those infected with HIV.

—Steven F. Scheibel, M.D.

It was the early 1980s. I was looking forward to taking on the challenge of a post-doc fellowship in infectious diseases and was headed to Rochester, New York, for an interview at the University of Rochester Medical Center.

The day I met Bill Valenti, M.D. was cold, rainy, and gloomy, but coming from Chicago, I was familiar with "lake effect" weather. Bill sat cross-legged on his desk chair. He swiveled in the chair to face me and said he had a bit of a head cold. We had a conversation about our interests in infectious diseases and possible research interests—typical interview topics. But not typical was the easy rapport, the curious nature, the quick intellect, and the quirky sense of humor. I sensed a man with a mission and hoped I would have the chance to work with him.

When I arrived on the scene in Rochester for my infectious diseases fellowship, the hospital already had a burgeoning census of inpatients with opportunistic infections/HIV-associated cancers/AIDS. These were the bad times, with AIDS stigma affecting the delivery of humane healthcare. Indeed, the populations disproportionately infected with HIV—gay men, intravenous drug users, and minorities—were considered disposable by some, and thus, they reasoned, HIV would serve to purge society of these "undesirables."

As the onslaught of AIDS continued, there was a split between those who believed that patients with AIDS deserved quality healthcare, compassion, psychological/psychiatric services, specialty pharmacies, social services, housing, hospice, and hope. Others treated AIDS patients with disdain and disgust, denying them the level of care offered to HIV-negative patients.

Bill and I found ourselves in the middle of the controversy. Who was going to advocate for our AIDS patients so that they received the level of care commensurate with other members of the community? The clinical care of HIV patients was and has been provided by gay men, women, and minorities in large part. Others chose not to work with this population, often because of homophobia, racism, and fear.

As the situation worsened and the number of patients needing care escalated, we asked our colleagues to step up to the plate with us—a number of very devoted and fearless nurses, psychiatrists, social workers, pharmacists, and administrators joined together to work as a dedicated team.

And then we asked for the help of the community-at-large. The response was immediate, generous, and committed. Rochesterians, and those from the outlying areas, volunteered to help with their time and donations to support an all out war against an invisible virus that caused very visible, devastating consequences. It became de rigueur for there to be fundraising and special events; outreach; and individual and corporate donations to support our efforts.

Our lives became part of our work. Friends became patients and patients became friends. Our friends died, and we attended many celebrations of life. We united with minorities, those with addictions, the LGBTQ community, and many families of our patients to improve services for those with HIV/AIDS. Through these cooperative relationships, Community Health Network and AIDS Rochester were created to provide medical care and case management services for our patients.

Bill and I and a handful of gutsy nurses took charge. We mobilized our team—much like a MASH unit in a war setting—and went to work. There were no drugs, there was no research, there were no answers at first, so we treated opportunistic infections and spent long hours in the lab after clinic hours.

The AIDS epidemic would be a test of our spirituality. Many passed with superlative marks; others failed miserably. Starting as early as 1981, those who fought the AIDS epidemic organized and developed grassroots organizations that provided housing, food, medical care, HIV testing, bleach kits to sterilize needles and prevent spread of HIV and hepatitis C, hospice care, free legal advice, transportation, assistance with housekeeping, grocery shopping, and other services.

Grassroots organizations, like AIDS Rochester Inc. (ARI) and Community Health Network (CHN), which Bill and I founded, responded to the overwhelming need and provided safe and compassionate medical homes for patients and their families. At CHN, the concept of "one-stop shopping" was realized with the provision of comprehensive medical care, an on-site pharmacy, social services, mental health and addiction services, laboratory services, and multidisciplinary case management. One of the first such clinics outside of a hospital, it became the standard of care for many similar clinics that sprang up around the country.

These safe homes for those with HIV/AIDS helped organize patients to insist on better treatments. With the vital participation of AIDS activists, notably the AIDS Coalition to Unleash Power (ACT UP), the advocacy movement confronted and challenged the U.S. Food and Drug Administration, as well as the pharmaceutical industry, to gain faster access to newer, safer, and more potent HIV medications.

At first, the care for AIDS patients was primarily the treatment of opportunistic infections. These infections occur when the immune system is severely impaired. Since there were no HIV medications available at the beginning of the epidemic, the immune system remained crippled, causing patients to suffer repeated episodes of these infections and leading to much suffering and agony which was only relieved by death.

AZT was the first anti-HIV medication available in 1987—two years after the HIV antibody test became commercially available. That's six long years without medication. Subsequent medications were administered individually during the era of single-drug therapy (monotherapy).

With the advent of other HIV medications, we learned that dual combinations of HIV medications prolonged the period of HIV suppression and immune system restoration beyond that of monotherapy. However, with time, most patients became resistant to these dual medication combinations.

The real turning point in the AIDS epidemic was the treatment with at least three HIV medications in combination. Initially, this was thought to be the cure, but it was not. After I left Rochester, I continued to do HIV care in San Francisco. My longtime collaborator, Dr. Brad Saget, and I presented our experiences with the treatment of HIV with multiple drugs in combination and showed "durable and sustained" suppression of HIV reproduction; in other words, virus reproduction slowed down and stayed that way. This combination antiretroviral therapy became known as highly active antiretroviral therapy or HAART.

Still, three drug combinations ("AIDS cocktails") did not result in a cure. Saget and I hypothesized correctly that HIV remained integrated within the human chromosome and is the source of re-seeding HIV infection once HIV medications are discontinued. Those cells that have HIV genetic material integrated within the human chromosome can have little or no evidence of HIV proteins on the surface of the cell. These cells represent the reservoir of HIV infection and are the source of low-level HIV replication and ongoing inflammation. This causes the premature onset of many diseases associated with aging and continues to plague our HIV-infected patients to this day.

Still, this era heralded many important advances, including prevention of mother-to-child transmission of HIV infection and also treatment as a means of preventing transmission of HIV infection to HIV negative sexual partners. With more potent and tolerable HIV medications available, patients were better able to take HIV medications on a daily basis. Single-tablet regimens (STRs) further helped to streamline treatment to one pill once a day.

Other advances include post-exposure prophylaxis (PEP) for those with occupational exposures (e.g., needlestick) or after condomless sex that use HAART to prevent infection. Pre-exposure prophylaxis (PrEP) is a further advance for preventing infection in HIV negative people due to sexual exposures. With a pill a day (and safe sex practices), sexually active people can be protected from contracting HIV.

In 35 years, we have moved from an incurable disease to a chronic disease and now to a potential world without AIDS. New York State has established a goal of reducing new HIV infections below epidemic levels by 2020—the End the Epidemic by 2020 initiative.

While vaccine research continues, there is ongoing research for a "functional cure." A functional cure is when after some interventions, the result is no HIV activity after discontinuation of HAART. Only one such cure has been documented so far. This occurred in a patient with leukemia who was treated with chemotherapy, radiation, and bone marrow transplants. However, the donor bone marrow was naturally resistant to HIV infection, making the patient's immune cells resistant to HIV infection. We all await further "cure" efforts that are affordable to the millions of HIV-infected people all over the world.

Bill and I are still among the legions of workers who care for those infected with HIV. We have survived our own health crises and lived to tell about them.

Steven F. Scheibel, M.D.
Palm Springs, California
February 2017

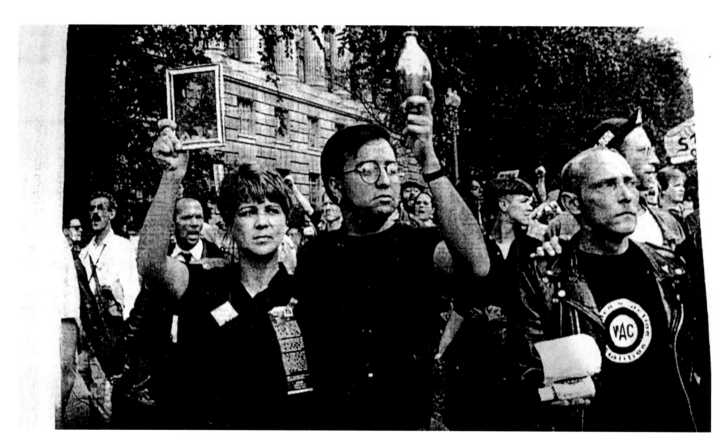

▸ War Games. Community Health Network staffers Lisa Brozek, nurse, and Ken Maldonado, development director, at a Washington, D.C., protest. The group spread the ashes of people who had died of AIDS on the White House lawn.

PROLOGUE: WAR GAMES

What's past is prologue.

—William Shakespeare, *The Tempest*

In terms of AIDS, what's past is indeed prologue. Shakespeare said it first in *The Tempest,* only under different circumstances.

Today, 35 years after the first case of AIDS was described, we talk about ending the HIV epidemic by 2020. To understand what it will take to bring new HIV cases below epidemic levels, we need to know how we got to this point.

This book is for the record. It is my effort to document the early era from the first case reports in 1981 through the advent of combination HIV drugs in the early 1990s. The so-called three-drug "cocktail," officially known as highly active antiretroviral therapy or HAART, was transformative. The term HAART was an important part of the vernacular of the era.

Today, all of the HIV drugs in common use are potent or "highly active." The approval of the HIV viral load test in 1996 helped us understand whether HIV drugs were working or not. That test helped to make HIV a chronic, more manageable disease.

In the early years, we never imagined we would reach a point where we could talk about ending the epidemic. It was a different era. So many words spun around in our heads while we tried to make sense of what they meant and how they fit together:

Body fluids, health crisis, incurable illness, the epidemic, pandemic, AIDS crisis, death sentence, AIDS hysteria, the virus, lymphadenopathy-associated virus (LAV), high-risk groups, safe sex, safer sex, injection drug use, hemophiliacs, Haitians, AIDS babies, children with AIDS, women with AIDS, transfusions, occupational exposure, antibody test, gay-related immune deficiency (GRID), AIDS-related complex (ARC), gay plague, AIDS victims, pneumocystis pneumonia, inhaled pentamidine, dextran sulfate, AL-721, Compound Q, Kaposi's sarcoma, cryptosporidiosis, molluscum contagiosum, hairy leukoplakia, thrush, lymphadenopathy syndrome, AIDS wasting, and the ACT UP advocates' signature: "Silence=Death."

My patients. Each one of them, in ways small and large, taught me something about the human condition. It has been a privilege to be their doctor.

My colleague and Community Health Network's (CHN) head nurse, Carol Williams, quoting Charles Dickens, said recently, "It was the best of times, it was the worst of times." She was right; it was both.

We experienced the *best of times* when community people rose to the occasion to get involved in some way. The epidemic forced us to think in new ways, combined the art and the science of medicine in the best interest of patients, put condoms on the map, brought discussions of sex and sexuality front and center, linked

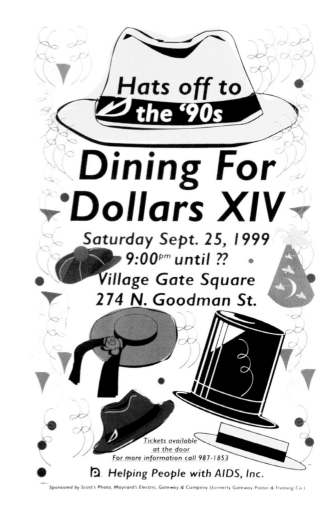

▸ By 1999, Dining for Dollars was raising $100,000 a year for local AIDS organizations.

the community together, and took gay rights, women's rights, advocacy, access to healthcare, and empowerment to new levels.

By 1986, there were 10,000 cases of AIDS reported in the U.S. The fatality rate was 75 percent. That same year, Jackie Nudd, executive director of AIDS Rochester, and I went to Auburn State Prison to do an educational program for prison staff. Almost 200 cases had been reported in New York State prisons by that time. Condoms weren't allowed, so we couldn't talk about sex in prisons. We promoted HIV testing, but testing was complicated in the corrections system, and it would be another year before AZT would be available. They served us lunch for our efforts. It's true what they say about prison food.

Also in 1986, 101 new cases of AIDS were reported in Rochester. The HIV antibody test had been approved a year earlier, and there were 200 patients in care in the Strong Memorial Hospital clinic. As the number of patients in the clinic began to increase, I met with Dan Meyers and Jerry Algozer, two friends and community leaders. I asked for their help raising money for patients. "Of course," was their answer, and they went to work, mobilizing their social networks. The result was "Helping People with AIDS" (HPA), a fundraising group that, over the next 17 years, would raise more than a million dollars for patient care. It would be another four years before any real federal funding for patient care was available through the Ryan White Care Act, so we were desperate. Also, this was before social media had a grip on us, and we relied on conventional media and word of mouth to promote our efforts.

The HPA concept was simple. People hosted dinners in their homes, and then the guests converged on one place for the after-party of dancing, drinking, entertainment, and dessert. We held the first event at the Village Gate and created a nightclub vibe with low lighting and black plastic trash bags covering the concrete columns. It was beautiful; only later did we realize that the fire marshall would have closed down our important event as a fire hazard.

We had no idea if this first AIDS fundraiser would work. We knew we had a hit on opening night when Dan Meyers and I peeked outside and saw a line of people down the block waiting to enter. Inside, I knew we were on track as I stood in a corner of the room, listening to the band, and watched the dancing skills of Richard Sarkis "dip" the black-sequined Diane Chevron.

Deemed a tremendous success, this first event raised $39,000. Later, HPA would be led by Craig Nenneau, Bob Lebman, and hundreds of volunteers. HPA had no paid staff. Eventually, "Dining for Dollars" became a $100,000 annual event when it was held at downtown Rochester's old Midtown Plaza. Over those 17 years, thousands of people participated and did something about AIDS. HPA helped pay for medication before federal funds were available, created a wish list for patients, and saved lives.

Jeff Kost, a community member, had just launched his career in his family's retail business. He described how volunteerism grew organically in the 1980s and became an essential response to the urgent needs of friends and families. He spoke of how the feeling of helplessness, in the face of the sickness and death of friends, inspired him to get involved with HPA and other AIDS activities. Later, he would leave the family business to follow Jerry Algozer as development director at AIDS Rochester.

Today, the HPA archives, thanks to Tim Tompkins, who led HPA in its last 5 years, and LGBTQ community historian Evelyn Bailey, are housed at the Smithsonian's National Museum of American History. At the transfer ceremony in Rochester in 2012, the museum's archivist described the collection as an example of the grassroots efforts growing out of the LGBTQ community in the 1980s in response to the AIDS crisis.

What was the *worst of times* during the early days of the epidemic? AIDS gutted a generation of people. Patients died. Lives and careers were interrupted. Families were in turmoil. A new kind of stigma emerged. Fear of contagion. Homophobia. At one point, it seemed as though all of my patients were 32-year-old men who were facing death.

The social climate of the era waxed between benevolence and cruelty. The death of a partner from AIDS called into question a whole series of relationship and grieving issues that had not been seen before on such a large scale.

The loneliness experienced by some patients was compelling. Survivors often didn't do much better. I saw many episodes of family members wanting to rid themselves of the surviving partner. There were squabbles over wills, real estate, bank accounts, and household goods.

Validation of gay relationships was on shaky ground in those days; hopefully, it will be less so today with marriage equality. One of my patients went into therapy after his partner of eight years died. He was overwhelmed by sadness. He thought that he could weather the emotional storm until the partner's parents told him that he was not welcome at the funeral and that he would have to move from the house they shared for 10 years since it was owned by the deceased.

There was no will leaving the house to the survivor. "Not only have I lost my partner and best friend," he told me during one visit, "but I lost my home." The bickering back and forth over possessions also became a huge distraction from the surviving partner's healing. He wasn't allowed to grieve peacefully.

The contagion wars were no better. Fear of contagion drove people into a frenzy of irrational behavior and thinking. There were calls to quarantine people with AIDS and efforts to outlaw gay bathhouses, gay bars, and adult movie theaters and bookstores. Jackie Nudd, AIDS Rochester's executive director, and others of us shot back and said those efforts would drive people underground and that education, outreach, and HIV testing were better alternatives. The discussions were endless, frustrating, and, at times, ugly.

For a time during the early years, I wore army fatigue pants, a black t-shirt, and combat boots around the house in the evening and on weekends. I remember telling Steve Scheibel that I needed to set the mood, even though it was totally out of character for me. We laughed about it, but deep down, we knew it wasn't funny.

Why the war games mentality? It helped cut the tension on several fronts. We needed a response to those who weaponized AIDS as a form of punishment. The medical war required us to think ahead, advocate for patients, and be aggressive. We never knew what decisions would need to be made when we went to the office each day. In fact, we learned to expect the unexpected, waiting for the other shoe to fall. We found ourselves in a thick fog of issues none of us had ever encountered; quick decisions to be made, patients sick and in crisis, and death everywhere. These were very long days.

The sense of urgency was constant and often overwhelming.

I had done media interviews in the past, but once AIDS hit, I found myself in front of the camera or a reporter, being photographed and quoted in the next day's newspaper or being filmed for the evening news. Unlike my previous limited media experience, I was now in the hot zone.

I tried to watch what I said and how I said it, knowing that my media mentor, Bob Loeb, medical center public information director, and my mother were both watching and reading. Bob's coaching on how to speak in sound bites saved me from falling into many a rabbit hole.

By the time Community Health Network, our HIV medical clinic, opened in 1989, almost 25,000 people in the U.S. had died of AIDS. CHN was poised to be on the forefront of the AIDS effort. Our early, aggressive "hit hard, hit early" mantra was gaining traction slowly. However, the final consensus for treating HIV patients as early as possible wouldn't be settled until 2013.

Lisa Brozek, CHN's clinic infusion nurse, said recently that the pace and devastation around her felt like a "war zone." She was right.

The pace was frenetic. Sid Metzger, CHN social worker, once said that she felt like a caged mouse, running on a wheel that never stopped.

Bishop Matthew Clark of the Roman Catholic Diocese set the tone for religious leaders in the effort. Recently, he quoted Pope Francis in reference to the era, saying that "the Church during a health crisis is like a field hospital during wartime."

Still, there were lighter moments. On some chaotic days at Community Health Network, we

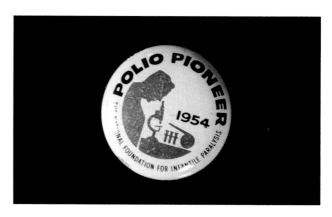

▶ Polio Pioneer lapel button.

would laugh at the irony and drama of it all. As Steve Scheibel said more than once, "I love this place when it sizzles!"

True to Shakespeare's past as prologue quote, my growing-up years provided a dress rehearsal for what I would confront many years later when the AIDS crisis hit.

I was a serious kid. I never went through a stage where I wanted to be a cowboy. I *always* wanted to be a doctor. My inspiration for a career in medicine was my great-uncle, Dr. James Chiappetta, my mother's uncle and a family medicine physician in the Public Market neighborhood of Rochester. Along with my parents and Dr. Jonas Salk, who developed the first polio vaccine, he was my hero.

When I was in high school, I had an assignment to interview someone whose occupation was the one I wanted when I "grew up." The decision was easy. I interviewed Uncle Jim. We sat in his exam room after office hours one day, and I asked the questions. I remember only the last question: "What does it take to be a good doctor?" His response was eloquent: "A genuine love of humanity." End of interview. I was on my way to a white coat and stethoscope.

Uncle Jim died in 2014 at the age of 107. Over the years, I have met many of his patients. They all say the same thing: "He was a fabulous doctor. He took care of our entire family. He made house calls. He didn't charge us when we were broke." Dr. Lawrence "Larry" Chessin, one of my early mentors as an intern who knew Uncle Jim from the staff at Genesee Hospital, once told me that he was a "fine physician of the old school" and a "real gentleman."

My parents had clear expectations that set the course for my life as well: save your money, work hard, pay attention in school, and be nice to people. Since I grew up in the polio era, we also learned how to wash our hands vigorously before eating and after using the bathroom. It seems like I've spent a good part of my life dealing with matters of contagion. My parents' hand-washing lessons would serve me well as Strong Memorial's hospital epidemiologist many years later.

The art of running a small business came from my wise father who ran a wholesale produce business at 16 Public Market in Rochester. We worked side by side for many years on weekends and summers. I was bored by the experience, thinking that I was cut out for greater things. He encouraged me in my career plan and told me more than once that I could do anything I wanted if I put my mind to it. At home, he tried to instill in me a love of classical music. As we filled plastic tubes of tomatoes on the packing machine conveyor, he would offer bits of advice. Many years later, I would put the pieces together and come to appreciate his strategic approach to business and life and his love of music.

We were fortunate to have a stay-at-home mother. An avid reader, letter writer, and news junkie, our mother was a constant presence during our growing-up years. My first "risk-benefit analysis" was as a second-grader when my mother, at the young age of 28, enrolled my sister Elizabeth and me in the Salk polio vaccine trial. She and Uncle Jim had caucused, and he reassured her that the benefits of the trial far outweighed the risks.

In research-nurse style, she explained that there was a chance we would get the "sugar injection," her words for placebo. The vaccine trial started, and she went to work with her daily rosary to ensure that we received the real thing.

I recall my classmates lining up in the school library for the three injections. In the vaccine trial, 623,972 schoolchildren across the U.S. were injected with the vaccine or placebo, and more than a million others participated as "observed" control subjects. The largest field trial ever conducted, the results were announced in 1955. The trial showed that the vaccine was 80–90 percent effective in preventing paralytic poliomyelitis.

When I was seven years old, I went with my mother to Sibley's department store in downtown Rochester during a March of Dimes campaign, the organization that funded Salk's polio vaccine work. An iron lung, a monster of a steel tube, was on display. One type of polio (bulbar polio) paralyzed your breathing. The iron lung helped expand and contract your lungs to help you breathe. And that's where some polio survivors were doomed to spend the rest of their lives.

What a cruel disease, I thought. In modern terms, living in an iron lung would be like spending your life in the confined space of a CT machine. I was alone in the room, and I tapped my knuckles on the cold metal cylinder. I can still hear its hollow, clanking sound.

At the end of the vaccine trial, wearing a big smile, my mother gave us the good news. Elizabeth and I both received real vaccine and not placebo. I can imagine the sigh of relief she felt when she read the morning paper, as she did every morning. Newspapers screamed in 6-inch headlines: "SALK'S VACCINE WORKS!"

Nice work, Mom. You saved us from the iron lung. We received lapel buttons that said "Polio Pioneers." After the trial was completed, polio became yesterday's news. Our two younger brothers, Jim and Richard, would never know a world with polio.

My new hero, Dr. Jonas Salk, left me with an indelible impression of the noble work of wiping out disease. Imagine your life's work resulting in preventing polio, the scourge of the day. Just imagine being a part of the eradication of a terrible disease.

I do. I imagine a world without AIDS. Every day.

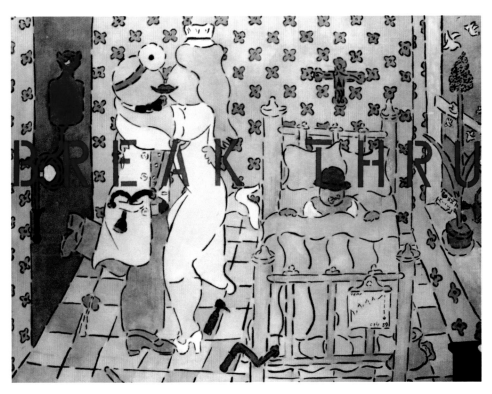

▸ *Break Thru*, William Nelson Copley, 1989.

Bill Copley, aka CPLY, (1919-1996) was a personal friend. His playful, energetic works are considered late Surrealist, a precursor to Pop Art.

In his prophetic words: "This painting is meant to express the spirit of hope and faith that the day of the AIDS breakthrough is surely coming."

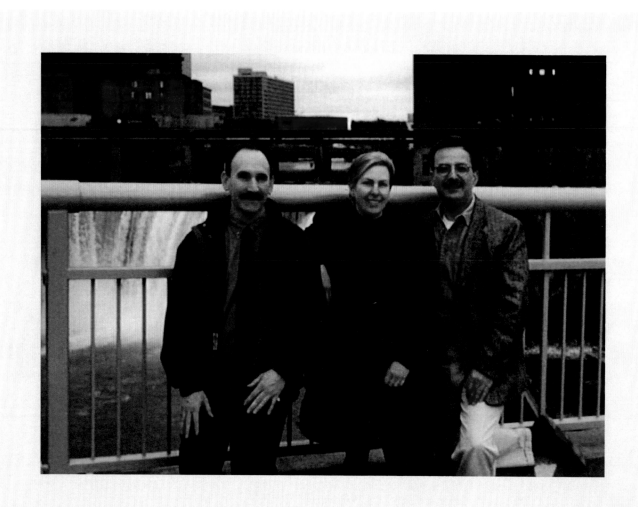

▸ Left to right: John Altieri, Sue Cowell, and Bill Valenti after an AIDS Task Force meeting, 1983.

1 | LEAD, FOLLOW, OR GET OUT OF THE WAY

The occurrence of pneumocystis in these five previously healthy individuals without an apparent underlying immunodeficiency is unusual. The fact that these patients were all homosexuals suggests an association between some aspect of a homosexual lifestyle or disease acquired through sexual contact and pneumocystis pneumonia in this population.

—Centers for Disease Control, June 5, 1981

June 5, 1981. I remember it very well: it was the day the Centers for Disease Control and Prevention (CDC) published its first report of five cases of pneumocystis pneumonia in gay men in Los Angeles and New York City. In those days, the CDC's *Morbidity and Mortality Weekly Report* came in hard copy. I read the report; then, rather than tossing it away, I created a file folder that I labeled "Infectious Diseases—Other."

I was intrigued by these cases. It was too early to call this a new disease, but still, I wondered what it meant. There was something unsettling about the patient descriptions. Even more interesting

CENTERS FOR DISEASE CONTROL

MMWR

MORBIDITY AND MORTALITY WEEKLY REPORT

June 5, 1981 / Vol. 30 / No. 21

Epidemiologic Notes and Reports
249 Dengue Type 4 Infections in U.S. Travelers to the Caribbean
250 *Pneumocystis* Pneumonia — Los Angeles
Current Trends
252 Measles — United States, First 20 Weeks
253 Risk-Factor-Prevalence Survey — Utah
259 Surveillance of Childhood Lead Poisoning — United States
International Notes
261 Quarantine Measures

Pneumocystis Pneumonia — Los Angeles

In the period October 1980-May 1981, 5 young men, all active homosexuals, were treated for biopsy-confirmed *Pneumocystis carinii* pneumonia at 3 different hospitals in Los Angeles, California. Two of the patients died. All 5 patients had laboratory-confirmed previous or current cytomegalovirus (CMV) infection and candidal mucosal infection. Case reports of these patients follow.

Patient 1: A previously healthy 33-year-old man developed *P. carinii* pneumonia and

▸ The Centers for Disease Control's first reports of AIDS, reported by Dr. Michael Gottlieb.

---

was the notation at the end of the report. Dr. Michael Gottlieb, a UCLA immunologist, reported the cases.

Michael had been a University of Rochester medical student and internal medicine resident. I recalled him rotating on the infectious diseases inpatient service with me, and he was bright, talented, and energetic. Although I didn't realize it at the time, our relationship had just changed. My former student had become my teacher. We would reconnect many times over the ensuing years as the AIDS story continued to unfold.

As I thought about these cases, I had no idea of the significance of his report or how it would change the course of history and our lives. "Who knew? We had no idea of what was to come," said Dr. Hannah Solky, a pediatrician-turned-psychiatrist who would later conduct a support group for the hospital clinic and, later, Community Health Network staffs.

Having just finished my infectious diseases fellowship, I was the hospital epidemiologist, the hospital's "disease detective," if you will. I did double duty in the University Health Service (UHS) as the assistant director for occupational health. Most of the work was medical center employee health and was infectious diseases-related, so it all fit together.

The job involved problem-solving and an understanding of how infections are or are not transmitted. It hit me one day while driving. The infections that the CDC was reporting were transmitted in a similar fashion to hepatitis B— through sex, blood, and needles and not by saliva or tears. It didn't take a great genius to figure this out, either. I was merely putting disease patterns together, the infectious diseases specialist's standard operating procedure.

In 1981, the hepatitis B vaccine was introduced. So, I sat back and continued to focus my attention on a hepatitis B vaccine program for Strong's healthcare workers, the infection control initiative of the moment. I saw patients on the inpatient service at Strong Memorial and was the eager junior faculty member, passionate about the responsibility I had been given in my new role as hospital epidemiologist.

By 1982, as I was getting my head around matters of the contagion of hepatitis B versus AIDS, a clinic for gay men was under way two floors below in UHS. One of our infectious diseases fellows, Dr. Tom Rush, and UHS nurse practitioner Sue Cowell had begun a screening program for gay men at risk for HTLV-III, the original name given to what we now call HIV. Tom Rush described the experience as another activity where they were finding answers before they knew the questions.

Their study—screening gay men at risk for HIV—was a "one-off"; it could never be done again. When they published their results, they highlighted their unique study population from Rochester, a city without "endemic AIDS." In other words, HIV transmission was limited and had not gotten its grip in Rochester yet. The study subjects were at risk but unexposed to HIV for the most part. They concluded in this once-in-a-lifetime study, published in 1986, that the immune system abnormalities seen in people with AIDS were, in fact, due to HIV. It was a beautiful piece of work that can only be appreciated all these years later. There isn't a place on earth that does not have endemic AIDS anymore.

Sue Cowell continued the fight by founding AIDS Rochester on her front porch with a group of local activists in 1983. To support the urgent need, she persuaded local mover and shaker Tim Tompkins to join in, and he became a major sup-

"THERE ISN'T A PLACE ON EARTH THAT DOES NOT HAVE ENDEMIC AIDS ANYMORE."

porter, donor, and fundraiser for the new organization. Later, Sue was Monroe County's AIDS coordinator, serving as the point person for all county programming related to the epidemic.

Despite my workload upstairs in infectious diseases, I learned a tremendous amount quickly. I was encouraged to think creatively. Since the infectious diseases unit was a major virology center, it was only natural that I would become a virologist of some sort. I spent my research time trying to understand hospital-acquired viral infections, something that was not yet on anyone's radar screen, and it would serve me later when AIDS hit.

Later in 1982, about six months after the CDC report, we were at our weekly conference. A resident presented a case of a local man, originally from a Caribbean island, now on the hospital service. He had a bizarre collection of infections, including herpes simplex of the esophagus, pneumocystis pneumonia, and a cytomegalovirus infection. We had seen these infections sporadically over the years but never all in the same patient.

I was distracted, reading mail, as I listened to the presentation. Then someone around the table said, "This is like the cases that the CDC has been reporting." I looked up. No one spoke for a few seconds, but we all knew that something was happening. What the CDC had been describing in their early reports on AIDS was now in Rochester.

By this time, the CDC characterized "high-risk groups" for AIDS: Haitians, homosexuals, hemophiliacs, and heroin users, cruelly dubbed by some media people as the "4 H Club." The Haitian epidemic probably originated in Africa and was fueled by extreme poverty in Haiti, at least in part, and it killed tourism to Haiti in those early days.

Our patient with AIDS was a footnote to the crush of patients that would follow. Not long after the Caribbean patient, the first gay man with pneumocystis pneumonia was admitted to the hospital. He was a local business owner who, despite our best efforts, died.

Others soon made their way into the hospital emergency department or clinic—men caught off guard at the height of post-Stonewall liberation. The 1969 Stonewall riots were a pivot point in gay liberation. The Stonewall Inn, a gay bar in New York's Greenwich Village, was the site of several days of riots between LGBTQ people of New York and the police. The result was the gay rights movement. After the Stonewall riots, activist groups were formed to concentrate efforts on establishing places for gays and lesbians to be open about their sexual orientation without fear of being arrested. LGBTQ people were more visible after Stonewall, and the movement

would refocus many years later in response to the AIDS crisis.

Who could possibly have known that what had been lurking in West Africa since the 1960s would end up in Rochester, New York? We were in no way prepared, but we swung into action nonetheless.

Most of the early cases occurred in people who were travelers to New York City. For a while, I deluded myself into thinking that AIDS wasn't really in Rochester but was imported from big cities like New York and San Francisco. I was wrong.

It seemed like the stream of people coming into the hospital was never-ending. Everyday people, high-profile people, and personal friends were part of an avalanche of people in trouble. I had some visibility in the hospital in my infection prevention role, and then I started to do some media interviews about this new disease. Once I started to see AIDS patients, I began to define my role as an AIDS doctor. I wasn't the only person who swung into action, but personally and professionally, I felt the need to respond to the crisis.

Not everyone went to the emergency department seeking care. Some people came directly to my office. One day, a high-profile man I knew from his community work popped into my office, which was sparsely furnished with a desk, two chairs, a file cabinet, and some bookshelves. He was one of the first of many people to sit opposite me and tell me his story. As a young man, he experimented with injecting drugs. It was only for a short time, and it was a long time ago. He was 40 years old, his career was on the rise, and he was sick.

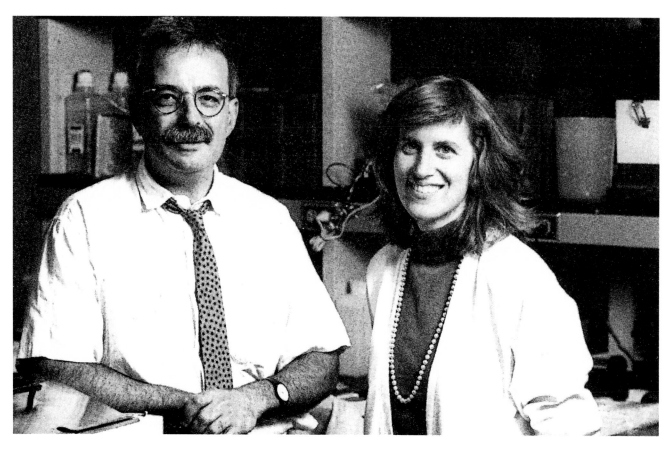

▸ Dr. Susan E. Cohn, an infectious diseases colleague of the era, and I met in the lab to discuss a trial using an HIV vaccine for treatment. 1994.

I began to realize the enormity of what was happening. Like many people who sat in those chairs after him, he was looking for a lifeline. During the conversation, he apologized to me for his past behavior. When he finished, we sat there in silence for what seemed like a very long time. I broke the silence and reassured him that he didn't need to apologize. I told him that he needed medical care, and we walked down the hall to the clinic and enrolled him as a patient. This experience established the connection between HIV and medical care for me and became my signature. At that point, I knew that my life had changed, and there would be no turning back.

Soon, I was given a lab assignment to try to stimulate the immune system's T-cells of people with AIDS; I was frustrated and getting nowhere. Ordinarily, when infectious agents challenge these cells, they respond and fight back. There was no response in the petri dish from the infection-fighting cells in my experiments. Impatient for results, I felt like a failure. What I did not appreciate at the time was that I had results. Those T-cells weren't responding as a result of HIV infection.

I worked on these experiments in the morning and tried to translate what I was learning when I saw patients in clinic in the afternoon. Then I had to translate everything that had gone on during the day into sound bites for the 6 o'clock news that evening. I was in demand with local media and learning the art of the sound bite.

I realized that I preferred working with patients and gave up on the lab work altogether. On the other hand, Dr. Steve Scheibel, an infectious diseases fellow at Strong at the time, was a lab jockey *extraordinaire*. He understood HIV from the patient level to the test tube.

We first met during his interview for the program and connected later when we all traveled to a national infectious diseases conference in Minneapolis. After a group dinner, Steve and I walked back to the hotel in the bitter cold. During that freezing walk, we broke the ice further and came out to each other. As we got better acquainted, we learned that we had common interests in gardening and cooking. After that, we would spend many afternoons and evenings discussing the AIDS crisis in his lushly planted garden.

A superb athlete and gymnast in high school, he is also a talented pianist and ballroom dancer. Steve grew up in the suburbs of Chicago and attended the University of Illinois, where he was

Phi Beta Kappa. We soon started to collaborate on patients, and he spent a lot of time in the clinic while also working in the lab.

I've always admired his deep understanding of the science behind what we were doing. In contrast to my "let's get it done" style, Steve often hit the pause button and stopped to reflect on the situation at hand. I imagined the chemical formulas circulating in his mind as he explained the biochemistry behind a drug or the science behind some disease state or other. Somehow, he was always able to tie it all together and deliver superb care to patients. In fact, he seemed to have some of the answers before we knew the questions.

We arrived at the concept of early intervention for HIV from two different places, met in the middle, and somehow it all worked. We clicked and, in addition to a major collaboration for more than 10 years, we have a lifelong friendship.

In the early days of Community Health Network, Steve launched a research program. We conducted an FDA-approved trial of an early HIV vaccine for treatment and enrolled almost 200 patients. He would go on to collaborate with Dr. Brad Saget. Steve had a small lab at CHN where he worked on an early HIV vaccine made from the plasma of our patients who had high T-cell counts. Considering the desperation in 1989 and 1990, the vaccine made sense, and patients were interested and willing participants.

Steve recalls the era. "We all had the same mission: to treat our patients in the best possible manner. I was the alchemist—mixing antivirals, trying to make potent and tolerable cocktails for patients. Bill was the doc/manager/diva-boss who, after hearing about our schemes, would either approve or disapprove and then move on to making his famous pasta salad."

My brief time in the lab, plus watching Steve's mind at work and admiring his ability to translate his discoveries to patients, gave me a healthy respect for the role of laboratory science in scientific discovery. It also helped define my own role as a clinician, administrator, and research collaborator. Over the years, I would learn a tremendous amount of science—and a few dance steps—from him.

By the way, I still follow a few of our early vaccine recipients. Nearly thirty years later—they are doing fine.

WILLIAM M. VALENTI, M.D.

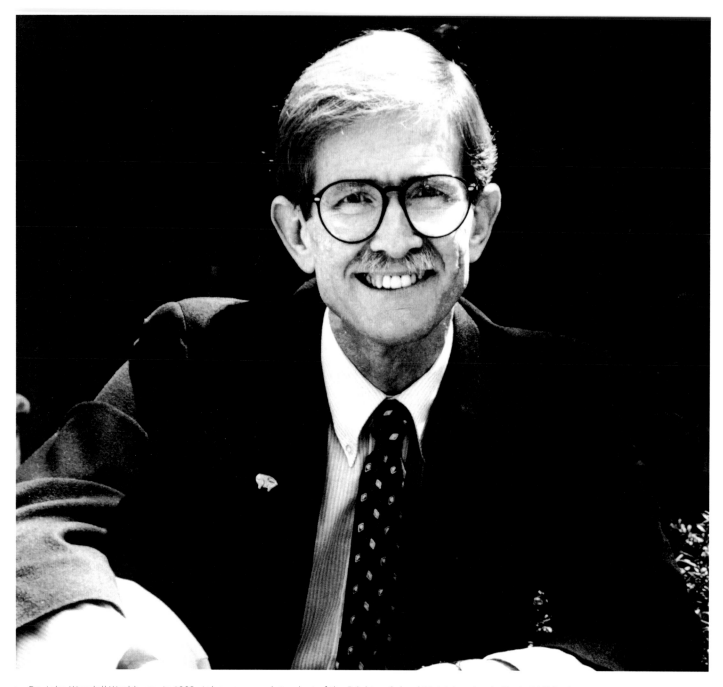

▸ Dr. John Wendell Washburn, Jr. 1983. John was superintendent of the Brighton School District and a dedicated AIDS educator.

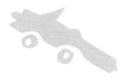

2 | PIVOT POINT: A NEW REALITY

*I soon realized that, like it or not, I was the AIDS doctor and
that I was being held to a different standard.*

I came out in 1981. My emergence as a gay man coincided with
the emergence of AIDS, a period of intense conflict for me. I needed
to be discreet and not give anyone a reason to include me in any
less-than-complimentary discussion. A friend once told me that
"your behavior should be above reproach." I listened to her.

I learned many lessons in the early years of my new reality—
lessons that have served me well throughout my career and my
personal life. These are just a few:

First, it was important to remember that Rochester is a very
small town. People talk. You've either gone to school with them,
you're related to them, you've done business with them, or you've
slept with them.

Reality: Actions speak louder than words.

Second, gossip was tempting but, more importantly, damaging and stigmatizing. Unless you were there, you have no idea of the real truth, so just sit back and listen. Don't pass it on.

Reality: My lips are sealed.

Third, my friends became my patients, and my patients became my friends. It would have been easy to become part of the "grapevine," but the second lesson saved me a lot of trouble. Besides, people trusted me, and I did not want to break that trust.

Reality: Tightrope walking is an acquired skill.

Last, confidentiality was critical, especially during the height of AIDS hysteria. I told my patients that what we talked about in the exam room was between the two of us. I said, "I don't discuss your personal information with anyone, not even my partner." Some people were surprised by this last part. But it was true: I never discussed patient information with him. Period. I still don't.

People shared their personal information and sexual histories with me in great detail. I listened and used what they told me to help shape the discussion of their healthcare. They told me these things in confidence and for a reason. They didn't want me to shake a finger at them.

Reality: I dropped the word "promiscuous" from my vocabulary.

Meeting People: My New Social Reality

In the days of my coming out, the dating scene was quite different from my previous experience. And quite different from dating in today's gay world.

We met up the old fashioned way—by socializing in gay bars on a Saturday night or Sunday afternoon, drinking beer, chatting people up, and hoping that something would happen.

Today, people meet digitally. Mobile apps are the "only way to meet people," according to a recent patient. At any rate, he forced me to think about how we communicate today. As I listened, I thought he was right. This is a different communication era; you can't send an emoji or a selfie on a landline.

Networking with friends of friends proved to be a good way for me to meet people. Susan Robfogel and I met when she was the hospital's legal counsel. She told me once that I should meet her new friend, John Washburn, the gay superintendent of the Brighton School District. She had met him shortly after he arrived in town from the New York area in 1981, and they hit it off immediately, she recalled recently.

A short time later, I met John the old fashioned way. I was at a social event, a very civilized party given by my landscaper friend, Craig Nenneau, in the garden he designed at a grand house on Douglas Road in Rochester. Craig would go on to be a fundraising force with the "Helping People with AIDS" group. Later, he started a men's support group at CHN. Craig, his sister Anne, and his mother Nelma became huge allies in the fight.

Back to John Washburn. I perceived him to be a man-about-town before I met him. As the party was winding down, I was standing alone in the garden loggia, lost in thought about something or other. I can still see his smile and feel his confidence as he approached me and introduced himself. If anything, in those days, I lacked confidence. New to the scene, I wondered if I would ever have a group of friends.

The intoxication I felt in the moment was a combination of John's charm and the mint

gardenias in bloom in the garden. We went back to his house that afternoon. Part of the house tour included his closet of several hundred pairs of Western boots. He always wore boots, even with a suit.

He introduced me to hundreds of people and opened my eyes to my new world. Bigger than life, John was a take-charge guy. I admired his intellect, confidence, razor-sharp wit, the laughs, his style. And, he was a *raconteur* like no other. Most of all, I admired his insight about people. His analysis of people in our network was impressive. He was always thoughtful, analytical, and right on target. John, six years my senior, became my mentor, my lover.

His wisdom came out in countless conversations. Every conversation was rapid-fire and a brain challenge. I remember sitting with him in front of the fireplace in the living room of my newly established East Avenue apartment. We were engaged in conversation in quiet, calm tones, talking about the events of the day. I said something about how I was "just so busy." His eyes lit up as he responded with a quick, patient smile. In a voice imitating the comedian Paul Lynde, he said, "Do you know ANYONE who isn't busy?" I knew then I had entered a new world. Hopefully, my own history as a middle-class overachiever would carry me through these new adventures.

But, there was a harsh reality to this new world of 1982. It was only a year earlier that I had my epiphany while reading the CDC report of the first cases of what was now known as AIDS. At this point, our formerly low-key infectious diseases clinic had become the AIDS clinic. My patients' stories were all very similar: extensive travel histories to exotic places, meeting men, and hooking up. New York City travel was the ground zero of their sexual histories.

I began to fear for my safety and for the safety of my friends and my patients. I began to fear for the safety of everyone. I lost my boundaries early; my social life soon became my work life. Somehow, I managed to maintain my social calendar, be in the office on schedule, and keep up with my increasingly heavy travel schedule to give presentations on AIDS.

John continued to help me expand my network of new friends. He introduced me to Dan Meyers whose fundraising prowess would later be pivotal in our local fundraising efforts. Another of John's contemporaries was Wally Miller. Wally, a consummate host, entertained

"THINGS HAD CHANGED. WE JUST DIDN'T KNOW IT YET."

his wide circle of friends regularly at his new, modern house on a peninsula in Irondequoit Bay. A lively personality, Wally was good to his friends with his hospitality, beach club vibe, endless open houses, and groaning food table.

I remember one gathering at Wally's. It was a hot, sticky Saturday evening with 50 or so men in his pool, screaming, laughing, and carrying on like high school boys. In the midst of the hijinks, I had an uneasy feeling that something was about to change.

Later on, it hit me. *Things had changed.* We just didn't know it yet.

WILLIAM M. VALENTI, M.D.

Task force on AIDS is formed in Monroe

A Monroe County task force on AIDS, the devastating disease that destroys the immune system, has been formed to coordinate care for patients and to educate the public.

Ten cases of AIDS, with three deaths, have been reported by local physicians. Nationwide, health officials have charted 2,577 cases and 1,072 deaths.

The task force, formed by the state Health Department, is being chaired by Dr. William Valenti of the University of Rochester Medical Center and Jackie Nudd, president-elect of the Gay Alliance of Genesee Valley. The alliance provides medical referrals, speakers and an AIDS hotline.

The task force hopes to expand that hotline to 24 hours, along with planning educational programs. It also will address the needs of potential or diagnosed AIDS patients, such as screening procedures and long-term care outside the hospital.

"There is a lot of misinformation or incomplete information (about AIDS)," Valenti said. "One of the goals of the task force is to get accurate information to the general public as well as the high-risk groups."

Those likely to contract AIDS are homosexual and bisexual men, Haitians, present or past intravenous drug users, and hemophiliacs.

The task force will be submitting proposals for part of the money New York state is allocating for AIDS educational and research programs. The Legislature has set aside $5.25 million, including $600,000 for community groups.

About 20 members of the task force, representatives of various health organizations, met this week, Nov. 15, Valenti said.

▸ *Democrat and Chronicle,* November 3, 1983. Trouble in paradise. By 1983, when the local Rochester Area Task Force on AIDS was formed, there had been ten cases of AIDS and three deaths reported. This was the beginning of the local epidemic.

15

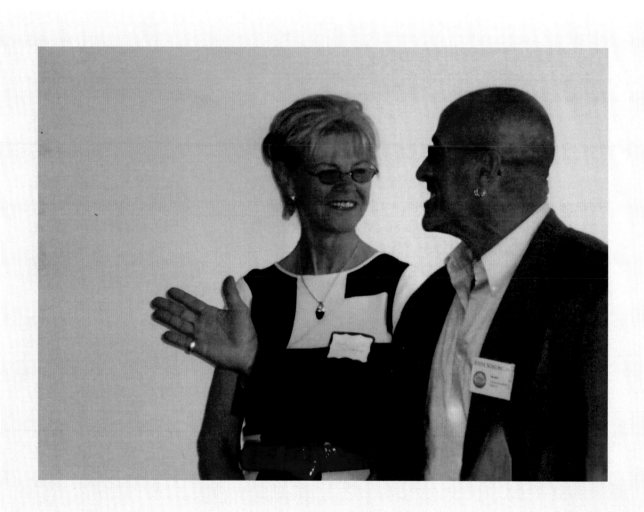

▶ Carol Williams and Steve Scheibel are having an animated discussion at Community Health Network's 20th anniversary celebration, 2009. Steve is telling Carol about his latest research discovery. Carol shows the same understanding smile that she had many years ago when I told her I was gay.

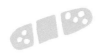

3 | THE CHIEF NURSE: CAROL WILLIAMS

It was the best of times, it was the worst of times.

—Carol Williams, quoting Charles Dickens

Carol Williams was organized, efficient, and passionate about the work. We first met when she was a staff nurse in the hospital outpatient clinic where we saw our AIDS patients before the infectious diseases clinic was established in its own space.

I was coming out as a gay man at the beginning of the AIDS crisis and keeping it to myself. Carol and I were having a cup of coffee in the staff cafeteria one day, and I blurted out, "I want you to know—I'm gay." With her beautiful smile, she said, "I know." It was at that point I knew we were on solid ground and that she could read my mind.

Today we talk about working at the "top of your license," meaning someone works at the maximum that their professional license allows. Carol did. She eventually joined the HIV program and quickly became a skilled clinician in her role as a clinical trials study nurse.

By 1988, when we were talking about what would soon become the Community Health Network, the decision as to who would be our head nurse was a no-brainer. Carol played a pivotal role in getting CHN established and running. In addition to starting from scratch to get us ready for our New York State clinic license by the health department, she became the general contractor on the clinic build-out.

The landlord was going to reconstruct the space—the former Elk's Club bowling alley on South Avenue. Overseeing the process was difficult for me—the endless meetings, the level of detail, and the delays were well beyond my expertise and comfort zone.

Carol and her family had just moved into a new house, and she had recent experience with buildings and contractors. One day I asked her to be the general contractor on the clinic project. She accepted graciously and without any obvious hesitation. Once she took on this role, we were on track.

She knew what we needed to do and made it happen. For example, she was determined to find a way to prevent and treat pneumocystis pneumonia with the drug, inhaled pentamidine. This treatment was usually done wherever the equipment could be squeezed in. In our ahead-of-the-curve model, we decided that CHN would have a pentamidine room to meet the demand. Carol's job was to create something that didn't exist anywhere else.

"I remember working with pulmonologists from around the country trying to design a negative-pressure pentamidine treatment room. We were so desperate for an organized approach to manage all of the pneumocystis we were seeing," she said recently. The final design consisted of a room with four separate booths so that we could treat several people at a time.

The negative-pressure system that she designed worked and passed the health department inspection with no questions asked. Instead, they gave kudos to Carol for her work putting the whole thing together.

Carol was a remarkable clinician. She would later obtain her master's degree and become a nurse practitioner. But for the time being, she was our head nurse, CHN's majordomo. Carol was good at what she did. Very good, in fact. Our patients loved her because she offered a value-added component of a nursing background combined with clinical care. She was also a wife and mother, and that came out in her care of patients.

Carol spoke of one of our earliest patients, a young man with Kaposi's sarcoma, a cancer seen commonly in AIDS patients in the early days. He was in the hospital, near the end of this life. "It was before we even knew how the disease was transmitted. I was making hospital rounds, and I remember being in a white lab coat. This young man was from the Midwest, had been rejected by his family, and was all alone. He looked up at me and said, "Carol, I need a hug." I thought, I only have a lab coat on, I have three children at home. I hoped I couldn't catch this disease by hugging. It was one of those walls you climb over or walk through. I hugged him. What an incredible experience."

This was one of those dark deaths—patients alone and rejected by their families. Carol's experience with this patient was one of many thousands of such situations played out all over the world. While many families rose to the occasion to care for their loved ones, others did not. We saw this scenario many times over the years. It was heartbreaking to watch and only added to the helplessness that was all around us.

Family dynamics created additional conflict with gay couples. Another of our earliest patients died and left a partner of 15 years. They lived comfortably, and his partner was his caregiver until he died. The patient's family asserted their legal right to manage the dead man's affairs. The locks were changed on the doors of their house and the partner was homeless. The partner survived for a while, but he couldn't cope. He later committed suicide despite our best efforts to guide him through his new reality. The collateral damage of the era was harsh and overwhelming, at times brutal.

It's hard to describe the intensity of the relationships that developed between our patients and staff. We all had our own most memorable patients. Carol recalled one patient—a young woman, a local college student.

"I think I became a mother figure for her. She came from Africa and was separated from her family. She brought me a gift once that I have to this day. I remember we suggested she go to AIDS Rochester to attend a support group there. She told me later that while she was sitting in this circle of white, gay men, she told the group that she felt out of place as a black, heterosexual woman. One of the men in the group leaned over and said to her, 'Don't worry, honey. We're all girls here.' I remember one of the men in the group took her to a dance—dressed up in a tux and sneakers.

"As her condition worsened, she was admitted to the hospital. When I saw her one morning, she lay in the bed with two chest tubes. She murmured, 'You know what I'm grateful for, Carol?'

" 'No. What, honey?'

" 'I'm glad I don't have three lungs.'

"Her friends in the AIDS Rochester circle rallied around her and made stained glass sun catchers for the windows in her hospital room. When her family visited, I held her hand while I told them about their beautiful daughter—that she was dying, and why. These are things you do not forget."

I asked a lot of Carol—constantly. "Carol, can you … ?" or "Carol, I need … " Whatever the matter at hand, she always maintained her composure and sense of humor. Her response, with a devious, all-knowing smile, would often be, "I am here to serve." Then she would get it done. I co-opted that response and have used it thousands of times over the years.

In addition to seeing patients, Carol led the New York State approval process for Community Health Network. The "Article 28" license, referring to the part of the state health code that licensed hospitals and clinics, was daunting.

We were establishing a licensed clinic from scratch with policies and procedures to be written and the need to meet page after page of other health department requirements. Carol was faced with the additional task of balancing the regulations under our license with our need to be aggressive with treatment and still play by the rules.

"I remember preparing for the state license approval with the health department," Carol recalled. "I had written all the policies and procedures that I thought we would need. Then the health department people would come up with another request. I would ask them for details so I could locate 'that particular document.' They would say they had no specifics but that they needed such a document. I would tell them to wait a minute and then run in my office and write a policy or procedure. Chuck Gearhart, our 'everything guy' would hastily type it up. They accepted them all. Nothing like a heading on a piece of paper to check all the boxes. Oh, those were the days."

Carol was thoughtful and analytical, in contrast to my approach to make a decision on the fly and do it now. There were times when she would put the brakes on and say, "Let's problem-solve this one. Sit down for just a minute," and we would discuss the issue at hand and figure it out.

Another of her responses was the time she reminded me of an important deadline. I said, "I've got it penciled in." Her response was a prophetic, "We are all penciled in, doctor!"

She recalled that one of her jobs was to "keep you and Steve out of jail." At CHN's 20th anniversary celebration, we finally came clean about the underground clinic we ran on Friday nights. When I told the story to the guests, she smiled. Later, she said, "I'm glad I didn't know about it at the time, but I'm glad you did it."

Modeling the extraordinary nurse that she was, she ended her recent note to me saying, "Being chosen for this work was an honor."

The honor of working with you was all ours, Carol. Your legacy lives on as the community health center, Trillium Health.

'You can't lie to them'

An AIDS victim anguishes for her children and herself

By Michelle Fountaine Williams
Democrat and Chronicle

Her two children, she has discovered throughout this ordeal, are smart. "You can't lie to them," she says from her wheelchair at Strong Memorial Hospital.

She has one of her many headaches, so her voice is weak and tired this day. But the maternal pride comes through loud and clear.

"My oldest has already asked me how sick I am. I just (said) that I was getting better. I just dodge the issue."

Perhaps she doesn't tell her children the truth because she doesn't quite believe it herself.

She has AIDS — a disease still generally believed to affect only homosexual men, intravenous drug users and hemophiliacs.

But she is none of the above.

She is among a small, yet growing number of AIDS victims: Those who have contracted it through heterosexual relations.

"Her story could happen to anybody," said her doctor, William M. Valenti, head of the infectious diseases unit at Strong and an expert on AIDS — acquired immune deficiency syndrome — an infec-

TURN TO PAGE **6A**

▸ *Democrat and Chronicle,* December 17, 1986. In this article, our patient describes her hometown experience and how she was stigmatized. Her health improved enough for her to make the trip to Disney World with her children. Note the use of the term "AIDS victim" in the story. After a time, the activist and medical communities were able to convince our reporter colleagues that the term "person with AIDS" or PWA was enough to tell the story.

4 | A CHRISTMAS STORY: AIDS, AZT, & DISNEY WORLD

People with AIDS are warm, compassionate human beings who have the same goals as all of us.

—Ann Zettelmaier Griepp, M.D.

I was on assignment in our newly formed HIV clinic at the hospital. It was 1987. AZT had been approved, and there continued to be a push for new drugs for treatment. There was an unprecedented public health response, with community people mobilizing to confront the epidemic and a "MASH-unit" mentality in the hospital daily, doing something that had never been done before.

The first woman with AIDS that I cared for was a young 35-year-old, a widow with two small children. She was unusual for the time, because she had heterosexually transmitted HIV. She came from about 60 miles away—every month—with her mother and her two kids. Her husband had died of AIDS two years before. Now she was sick. Of course, we put her on AZT, and it worked for quite a while. She gained weight, had more energy, and looked and felt better.

When AZT stopped working, she started to slide again, and we were out of options. I felt desperate looking into her sad eyes and thinking of those two kids playing in the waiting room. During one of our office visits, I asked her, "What would you do if you could do anything in the world?" Her sad face lit up. She didn't miss a beat. "Take my kids to Disney World," she said immediately.

I thought, "Why not?" In those days, we had very solid relationships with local media. They couldn't get enough of the AIDS story, and I was

"SHE SAID THAT HER CHILDREN KNEW NOTHING ABOUT HER ILLNESS; THEY JUST WANTED TO GO TO DISNEY WORLD."

always available and ready with a sound bite or a comment. Why not put the word out and try to raise some money for her? And that's exactly what we did.

The local paper's reporter on the medical beat and I had a nice working relationship. She was always telling me, "Give me an exclusive." I nicknamed her Lois Lane, and she was good-natured about it. So, we gave her an exclusive. She wrote the story of "Mary." After all, it was Christmas, and we needed to disguise the patient's identity.

The "Helping People with AIDS" fund was ready. Mary's family was ready too. And excited.

The story appeared in the morning paper during the week before Christmas on December 17, 1987. The story was all true and gut-wrenching to read. In the interview, she talked about how people in her small town laughed at her and made jokes about her. She said that her children knew nothing about her illness; they just wanted to go to Disney World.

At that point in my media interactions, I was still a little rough around the edges. In the interview, I ranted about the "disgraceful behavior" of her townspeople. I called for more compassion for people with AIDS—the same compassion that came when someone was diagnosed with cancer.

When I arrived in the office that morning, there was a stack of messages from various media outlets that wanted their piece of the story. As Christmas Day neared, the money continued to come in—more than $1,500. In fact, one man called and asked to deliver a check for $250 personally. He remains a donor to this day.

Around the same time, I did a monthly, live discussion on AIDS on WXXI, the local public broadcasting outlet. One Friday evening, I was paired with a representative from a local conservative group. One of the group's positions was that AIDS was divine punishment for homosexual behavior, so I swung into action, culture-war style. I had met him before; we had appeared on the air together, and we always disagreed on the issues. It was no different with this broadcast, the last segment of a yearlong series. I think we all felt the tension in the studio.

When we were off the air, the lights on the set were still on us, and the camera crew and moderator stood in back in the dark. For some reason, we remained seated and I said something like, "You were really hitting below the belt tonight. Your approach to the AIDS problem offers no solutions; it doesn't go anywhere."

He looked at me and listened. Then I started to overheat. To make my point, I shouted, "Why don't you do something productive for a change? If you're such a decent person, why don't you give me some money to send my dying patient and her children to Disney World?"

As I continued, the moderator and camera crew stood there, watching and listening in silence, as our zero-sum game unfolded.

He said, "If I give you some money, will you really give it to her?"

"OF COURSE, I WILL," I shrieked.

Then he did what any decent human being would do. He pulled out his wallet and handed me $50. I accepted the money, thanked him with a handshake, and we left. On the drive home, I thought about our unholy alliance. We were able to put the culture war on hold for a minute and find some common ground, even though our definitions of decency differed widely.

I added his donation to the fund, and after the holidays, Mary, her mother, and the two kids went to Disney World for a week. Airplane tickets, one of the best hotels in the park, expenses—all were covered by donations. When they returned, the morning paper did a follow-up story on the "Trip of a Lifetime."

At our next office visit, Mary was all smiles, basking in the glow of having done something so memorable with her children. Then she handed me an envelope with a Minnie Mouse decal inside. We laughed, and I told her I'd treasure it always.

I walked with her to the waiting room after the visit to say hello to her mother and the kids. It was nice to see them all smiling for a change. Her mother and I hugged, and they left.

Six months later, Mary was dead. Dr. Ann Zettelmaier, now Griepp, our program psychiatrist, was with Mary's family during their vigil around her hospital bed on her last day. She recalls sitting with Mary's young sons and the family early in the morning watching the sunrise. "The glorious shades of pink and gold made it clear that Mary was on her way to a good place and that all would be well here on earth," Ann said. We used some money in the HPA fund to help Mary's family pay for her funeral expenses.

Fast-forward to 2016: Recently, I was looking for something in the basement. There she was, looking down at me from the door of the laundry room—Minnie Mouse—right where I put her 30 years ago.

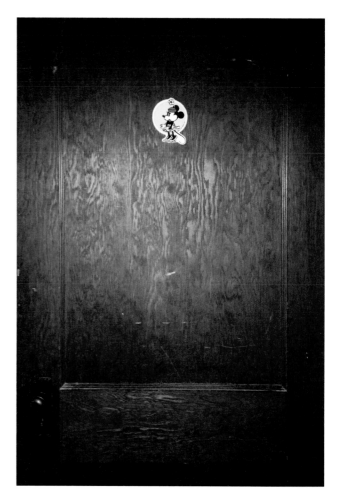

▸ There she was looking down at me from the door of the laundry room.

WILLIAM M. VALENTI, M.D.

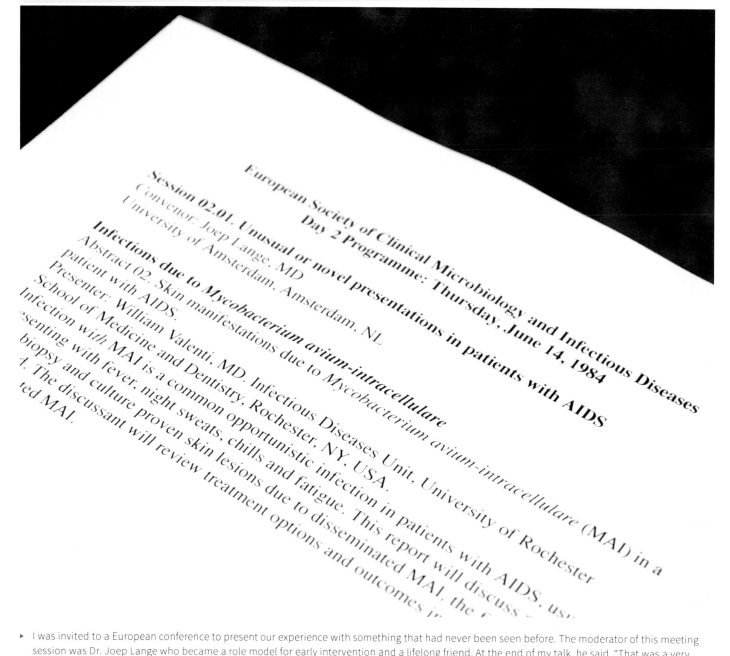

European Society of Clinical Microbiology and Infectious Diseases
Day 2 Programme: Thursday, June 14, 1984

Session 02.01. Unusual or novel presentations in patients with AIDS
Convenor: Joep Lange, MD
University of Amsterdam, Amsterdam, NL

Infections due to Mycobacterium avium-intracellulare
Abstract 02. Skin manifestations due to Mycobacterium avium-intracellulare (MAI) in a patient with AIDS.
Presenter: William Valenti, MD. Infectious Diseases Unit. University of Rochester School of Medicine and Dentistry, Rochester, NY, USA.
Infection with MAI is a common opportunistic infection in patients with AIDS, usually presenting with fever, night sweats, chills and fatigue. This report will discuss a patient presenting with fever, night sweats, chills and fatigue. This report will discuss disseminated MAI, the biopsy and culture proven skin lesions due to disseminated MAI, the ... d. The discussant will review treatment options and outcomes in ... ted MAI.

▸ I was invited to a European conference to present our experience with something that had never been seen before. The moderator of this meeting session was Dr. Joep Lange who became a role model for early intervention and a lifelong friend. At the end of my talk, he said, "That was a very elegant presentation." I was in awe of him. Often called a medical diplomat, he died in the crash of a Malaysia Airlines flight on his way to the 2014 International AIDS Conference.

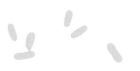

5 | 1985: AN AGE OF DISCOVERY

I knew that using steroids in a person with AIDS carried
some risk and that the evidence to support it was scanty.
I did it in desperation. I felt I had no choice.

Collaboration and Innovation

Before AIDS, pneumocystis pneumonia was a rare event, limited primarily to kidney transplant patients. During the early days of AIDS, pneumocystis became an everyday occurrence. One of my former medical students, Dr. Mark Stoler, led an effort that advanced the care for people with pneumocystis. Stoler, a young resident who later joined the faculty, would become our pathology department "go-to" person.

At the time, the entire medical center was responding at all levels to expand our capabilities to improve care for the increasing number of patients.

Stoler and a medical center lab scientist developed a new method of staining coughed sputum to identify the pneumocystis organism.

Their "discovery" took an older method of tissue staining and modified it to produce faster results. This early "rapid diagnostic test" eliminated the need for the more invasive bronchoscopy procedure for many patients. Bronchoscopy was the standard for diagnosis at the time and required a tube with a camera to get a piece of lung tissue, similar to the device used for colonoscopy today.

Using Stoler's new technique, we could diagnose pneumocystis pneumonia from coughed sputum, a true innovation for the era. I can still see us on our daily rounds in Mark's office, with the lights dimmed, peering into the microscope as we discussed our cases and confirmed the diagnosis on the spot.

Earlier diagnosis and treatment for pneumocystis pneumonia became our buzz phrase. My infectious diseases colleagues and Dr. Stoler were now joined at the hip.

I caught up with Mark Stoler recently. Now at the University of Virginia, he recaptured the collaborative spirit and energy of the era. "From 1982 to 1985, cases of AIDS started to increase rapidly in Rochester. Infectious diseases, pathology, microbiology, and hematology/oncology were interacting on a daily basis as we geared up to develop new technologies to support the demand."

Translating Discovery to Patients

Not long after this, we used Dr. Stoler's rapid test to make the diagnosis of pneumocystis.

I knew many of my patients personally. We had been following one of my friends in the clinic for a while. This was the era before we

"HE WAS STRUGGLING WITH THE VENTILATOR, AND HE WANTED YOU TO 'PULL THE PLUG.'"

knew that people with T-cell counts less than 200 were at risk for opportunistic infections like pneumocystis pneumonia.

He called one day saying he had a fever and was extremely short of breath, so I saw him in the E.D. He looked pretty sick, and his chest X-ray looked like classic pneumocystis pneumonia. We admitted him to the I.C.U. and, eventually, we put him on a ventilator, but he was still struggling.

Recently, Carol Williams reminded me about her "deal" with the patient. Her recollection speaks again to the bonds that we developed with our patients.

Carol said: "I got a call from you one day to come see a patient in the I.C.U. He was a friend of yours, a teacher, with pneumocystis pneumonia. He was struggling with the ventilator, and he wanted you to 'pull the plug.' "

I had been toying with the idea of giving him steroid drugs, even though the evidence for any benefit consisted of a few case reports from Europe. I checked in with Steve Scheibel, and he said in his usual style, "Do it!" I realized it was now or never. I wrote the orders and hoped for the best.

Dr. Hannah Solky recalled, "It seemed like you were always going against the grain."

Carol Williams recalled that these cases were always so hard on all of us. She sympathized with our patient that he was exhausted. Then she made a deal with him. We would sedate him and let him get some rest over the weekend. On Monday morning, we would remove the ventilator if he still wanted us to. That gave us a chance to administer steroids and observe him. At the time, this was unheard of, because steroids might suppress the immune system further. "A pretty gutsy decision," she said recently. She also recalled that some of my colleagues were skeptical of my plan.

During the weekend, I saw him on rounds twice daily. I remember sitting in the room at his bedside and talking to him and telling him that he could get better.

On Monday morning, bright and early, we went to see the patient. He was rested and breathing easier. We began to wean him off the ventilator, and he recovered enough to go back to teaching. The extra year of life was very meaningful for him and for us.

In 1990, a panel of experts weighed in on the matter and concluded that steroids had benefit in patients with severe pneumocystis pneumonia when given early.

Paris Breakthrough: So Much to Learn, So Little Time

I finally connected the dots a year later, in 1986, when I went to the second International AIDS Conference in Paris. A major report showed that people with CD4 T-cell counts under 200 were at risk for infections like pneumocystis pneumonia, and those patients should be given preventive treatment. As I listened to this presentation, I thought of this patient and how we might have prevented his pneumonia in the first place. I shook my head. It was like trying to get ahead of a fast-moving train.

I summarized the science of what we learned in an interview in the Rochester morning paper when I returned. The headline over the interview was "AIDS Breakthrough at Paris Conference."

The Patient's Story:
Science Versus the Subconscious

Hospital rounds on the HIV service were always lively and interesting. Dealing with all the unknowns around HIV challenged everyone's thinking.

After our patient in the I.C.U. woke up, I was talking to him on rounds with a few residents and students. He was breathing easier and sitting in a chair. During our visit, he thanked me for sedating him and recalled the deal with Carol. Then he talked about his experience on the ventilator.

He said that he recalled hearing my voice. He went on and said that all he could remember about the experience before he woke up was that everything was black and noisy. He had no recollection of what I said—only that he heard my voice.

As he was talking, I looked at my residents and students standing around his chair. Their eyes were riveted on him as he spoke. We listened to the patient in silence, with the constant, low-level "noise" of the I.C.U. in the background.

When we left the room, I quizzed the students on what the patient told us. There was no science to lean on here. We were in a parallel universe with this discussion. We concluded that, despite the absence of any science, talking to unconscious patients is a good thing.

Since that time, we have learned that studies of the brain waves of unconscious patients show a response to familiar voices. At the time, we could only speculate.

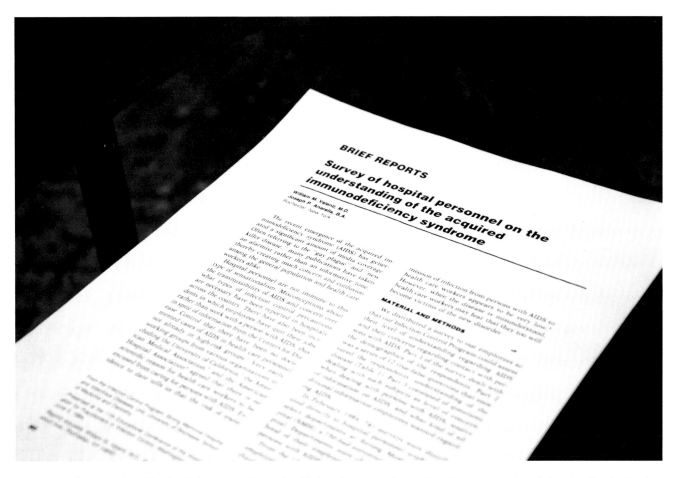

▸ Joe Anarella, a longtime friend, collaborator, and state health department mentor, and I wrote a paper on hospital workers' understanding of AIDS. Our conclusion was that hospital workers with patient contact understood transmission but were still anxious about it.

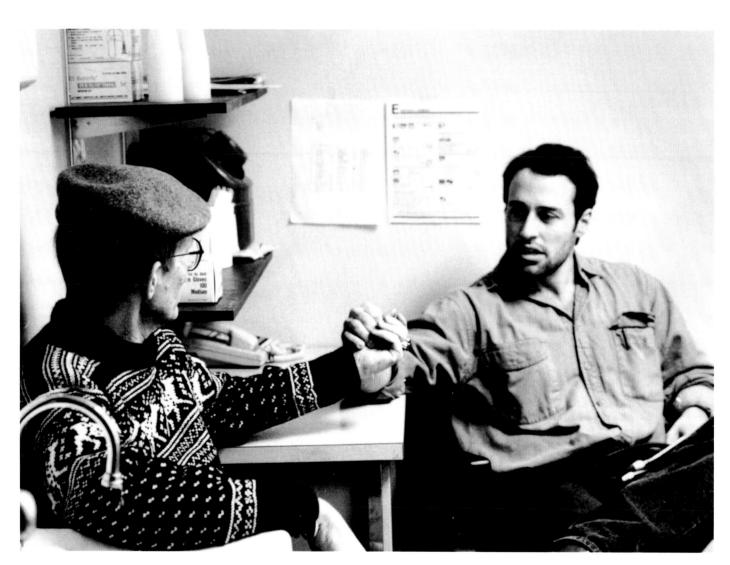

▸ Dr. Steve Scheibel and Dr. John Washburn in clinic sharing a moment. The patient is your friend and your friend is your patient.

6 | A PERIOD OF GROWTH

Always know your data, Valenti.

—Dr. Lawrence Chessin

The extraordinary John Wendell Washburn, a.k.a. Mona, was the first man I ever saw in drag. A group of us had gathered for dinner and socializing at his house one night. After we ate, Mona appeared wearing a gold lamé pantsuit, high heels, and a fancy hat—the works. The guests loved it! I had never seen anything like it.

John stood in front of me, leaned over, and looked in my eyes. Then he said, "Do you like it? It's just a little something I wear around the house," as if every Brighton housewife dressed like that. I was speechless.

All of this outrageous behavior was packaged during the day as the respected educator, Dr. John Washburn, superintendent of Brighton schools.

John's physician at the time was, coincidentally, one of my early mentors, Dr. Larry Chessin, an infectious diseases specialist, internist, and chief of infectious diseases at Genesee Hospital. Lawrence Norman Chessin remains a clinician, educator, mentor, role model, and friend today.

After a fellowship at the National Institutes of Health (NIH), Larry and his wife Rita returned to Rochester. Larry and I met when I was an intern.

One of the very early lessons I learned from Larry was the science of medicine. After I made a less-than-stellar case presentation to him on rounds one day, he reminded me, "Always know your data, Valenti." Understood, Larry.

Dr. Chessin also taught me that a very good infectious diseases specialist made a very good primary care physician. Larry always had lesbian, gay, bisexual, and transgender people in his private practice. When we discussed this once, he said, very simply, that people needed medical care regardless of who they were or where they came from.

During the early days of the AIDS crisis, our paths crossed in a more meaningful way.

Eventually, we would share John as a patient. Around 1983, John was in Genesee Hospital under Larry's care and had been diagnosed with tuberculosis (TB).

I recall my sense of relief that "it's only tuberculosis." After all, it was not AIDS, or so I thought. In my denial over John's health, I had ignored the possible AIDS/tuberculosis connection completely. Larry, on the other hand, was connecting the dots between HIV and TB in a different way, a connection that didn't exist at that point. During John's hospitalization, Larry called me and said, "We need to test him for the AIDS virus." I said, "We can't get the test. The only place they do it is at NIH."

Larry responded, "Then call NIH! Tell them I told you we need the test." I called his contact at NIH who agreed to do the HIV test as a favor to Larry.

John's HIV test was positive.

Larry and I (but really Larry) were one of the first anywhere to make the connection between tuberculosis and AIDS. The real understanding of the TB/AIDS connection would take another five years.

After about two years, John retired from the Brighton schools and came out as a man with AIDS. Larry used his media contacts to set up an interview for John that was conducted in Larry's living room in Rochester.

It was February 18, 1988. At the end of the day, I was wrapping up with Carol Williams in her office. She was poring over the evening paper when she looked at me and held up the front page. "Take a look," she said. "John Washburn is out." There he was—the superintendent of Brighton schools, the first high-profile person locally with AIDS, was out of hiding.

"I did it to put a face on all this," John would say later.

Carol and I looked at each other and nodded. "My, my, my," was all I could muster. I looked at the picture of John on the front page undergoing one of his treatments. The interview was compelling, as only John could do it. Determined to make a difference, John made a very brave, public disclosure. In those days, people with AIDS didn't reveal themselves. And here was John—out in the open, educating people, and fighting stigma.

By then, John's sister Patti Washburn had moved to Rochester to be his caregiver. My colleagues and I had become a part of the Washburn extended family and spent time with Patti, John's brother Jim, Jim's wife Suzanne, and the Washburn matriarch, mother Leota "Lee" Smith.

After he retired, John went on the road with his own AIDS education program and became a very popular speaker in educational circles. His talk was called "No More Broken Hearts." He was committed to educating young people about AIDS and thought that schools should play a central role in that education.

In his speech, he called AIDS "a sensitive and explosive topic." He alluded to "the best of times and the worst of times" from *A Tale of Two Cities* by Charles Dickens—only, he was referring to himself.

I remember helping him write the speech as his medical consultant. Quoting the CDC, he said that lives could be saved with education and that HIV could be prevented if we were "effective at teaching our children about sex and HIV prevention."

His friends were proud of what he was doing and often accompanied him on his trips when he spoke to major educational organizations. Most notable was a trip to New Orleans in March

1988. Dan Meyers and I were part of his entourage when he spoke to school board members at their national conference.

During this era, he founded the John Washburn Foundation. Its mission was to fund AIDS education.

John later moved to his adobe dream house in Santa Fe where he died in June 1989, six months after his 50th birthday. His time in Santa Fe was peaceful for him. Dan Meyers summed up John's healing in his remarks at John's memorial service in Rochester in August 1989. He said, "It would surprise the John Washburn of eight years ago when he entered this journey that the resolution of his inner tension is our biggest call to celebrate." Dan was correct. During his time in Santa Fe, the high-energy John became introspective and peaceful.

Ironically, he died as we were planning the Community Health Network, which would open a few weeks later, in July 1989.

I remember his 50th birthday party in Santa Fe in January 1989. As was his habit, it was a carefully planned series of events. Dinner and the birthday-cake reveal were at a restaurant, which was noisy and full of people. I watched as his mom, Lee, walked around the room, greeting the guests and trying to make conversation over the noise. When she arrived at my table, she was hoarse from talking. She took a cocktail napkin that was next to me and wrote, "Thank you." Then, she put her hand on my cheek and kissed me.

When he died, the assets of John's foundation were transferred to the Community Health Network where we created the John Washburn Library in his honor. I stood next to his sister, Patti Washburn, at the ribbon-cutting ceremony. As the local TV news cameras rolled, she cut the ribbon and said, "This one's for you, John."

I have many good memories of my friendship with John. And there is a room at Trillium Health where some of his personal items remind us daily of his courage and convictions. I miss him to this day.

In retrospect, Larry's referral to NIH was transformative for me. I had never made that kind of "cold call" before. After I made the call to Larry's NIH contact for John's HIV test, I grew up a bit more. I realized that there was no reason to procrastinate in this high-stakes game. People's lives were at risk.

I would never hesitate to call on people for help if it was in the best interest of the patient or the movement. The resources outside the system

"I REALIZED THAT THERE WAS NO REASON TO PROCRASTINATE IN THIS HIGH-STAKES GAME."

are there if you know who to talk to and how to do "the ask." The usual system of care works in its own way, at its own pace. However, an end run around it is necessary at times.

This early experience prepared me for the introduction of the HIV test that would finally be licensed in 1985. The original HIV test was an antibody test, and one of the concerns about testing was trying to understand what the results really meant. At the time, the argument was that antibody tests meant only that a person had been exposed to the virus.

If the test meant only exposure, then positive test results could be yet another means of stigmatizing people at risk, and we didn't need any more stigma. Many groups wanted to delay the introduction of the test.

What we didn't know until the test was licensed and in use was that a positive test also meant that the patient had the HIV infection. In other words, a positive test meant that you had the virus in your blood. When the viral load test to measure virus blood came in 1996, the meaning of a positive antibody test became very clear.

In early 1985, I found myself in the middle of the HIV testing war and out on another limb. Once the evidence was in, I couldn't ignore the link between HIV infection and virus in blood.

I went against the prevailing advocacy position, and prior to the test's approval in April 1985, I went public with my thoughts in support of the yet-to-be introduced HIV antibody test. My interview with the local newspaper was picked up by *The New York Times*.

I was quoted by name and institution as saying, "The HIV antibody test means that someone has HIV infection and virus in their blood. People who are HIV-positive need medical care."

A few days after the interview was published, a blizzard of mail arrived at the office. Apparently, ACT UP had organized a mail campaign, and I received almost 500 letters and postcards telling me that I was wrong and that testing would be harmful to people. Some of the mail was a little more graphic, but most merely admonished me for not fully thinking through the ramifications of testing.

Some time later, I met Michael Callen. Callen was an AIDS activist from New York. Diagnosed with AIDS in 1982, he was an early leader in our response to the epidemic. The Callen-Lorde Health Center in New York City is named in his honor.

He was an outspoken critic of AZT being used as a single drug. When we finally met at the state health department's AIDS Institute committee meeting, we found that we agreed about the need for more effective drugs, the painfully slow progress of drug development, and the lack of funding.

Michael advised me that he was behind the mail blitz. We laughed about the episode, bonded, and became friends after that.

In retrospect, I should have handled that one more diplomatically by reaching out to my advocacy colleagues and making it clear that I was talking about voluntary HIV testing only and not the mandatory testing that was being discussed by some people in irrational and frightening ways.

Instead, I dug in my heels. After all, it was a matter of urgency.

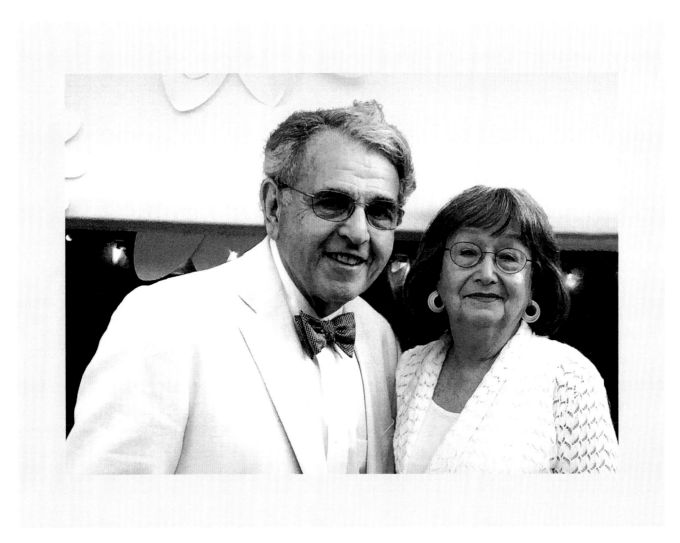

▸ Our friendship continues. Dr. Lawrence Chessin and his wife, Rita, at the Trillium Health White Party, 2016.

7 | THE NURSE AND THE NEEDLESTICK: AIDS IN THE WORKPLACE

Thankfully, transmission of HIV via needlestick to healthcare workers is a rare event. I have seen only one in my career.

We were doing hospital rounds on the HIV service when I was paged overhead. At the same time, my beeper went off from clinic. I called back and spoke to Carol Williams who told me, "They need you in E.D. There's been a needlestick. It sounds serious."

A staff nurse had backed into the needle during a cardiac arrest resuscitation attempt on an HIV-positive patient. She lost her balance and the needle went into her triceps muscle and hit bone.

I said to Carol, "Dig out that bottle of AZT you've been hoarding for a rainy day, and meet me in E.D." Her quick response, "I am at your service, doctor."

I entered the E.D. and was faced with a young woman sitting in bed, wiping tears from her eyes, explaining what happened. "I tripped. It was so crowded in there." Next to her was a young man stroking her shoulder.

Carol arrived. I could see the AZT bottle bulging in the pocket of her white coat. We inspected the wound. My heart sank when I saw the size of the hole. It was about a quarter of an inch in diameter with a visible tunnel. I nodded to Carol and she pulled the bottle from her pocket.

I explained to the nurse that the best chance to prevent HIV infection was high-dose AZT. I told the nurse that the sooner she started, the better. The young man, the nurse's fiancé, listened and nodded as I spoke. She continued crying, while Carol, in her motherly way, consoled her. Carol told her about the one month of treatment and possible side effects. Then she took the pills out of the bottle. Her fiancé agreed, and the nurse took the pills.

We saw her weekly in the clinic—then it hit the fan. Carol brought the news to me. "The lab just called. The three-week follow-up HIV test is positive."

The nurse had an appointment that day. We delivered the news. It was gut-wrenching. Her fiancé was with her, as he had been from the beginning. "We're getting married in a month," she told us. "What do we do now?"

They did indeed get married and had an HIV-negative baby within the year. Our nurse was courageous through the very rocky course of her illness. We continued to care for her until she died two years later.

When things began to settle down, we began to discuss whether the nurse should return to work in the I.C.U. or be reassigned to another area of the hospital. The discussions were complicated and emotional. There was no real precedent or guidance to help us.

In fact, we weren't the only employer dealing with the issue of AIDS in the workplace. In the 1980s, workplace contagion was a hot-button issue globally, because employees with AIDS were being assessed for fitness for duty in every industry.

In 1982, a friend, Ed Hubennette, was general manager at the Grand Hyatt Hotel in New York. When AIDS appeared, he dealt not only with employees who were ill and couldn't work but also with concerns about whether gay service staff should be working with customers. He describes the ripple effect globally that followed his career when he took a position with a hotel chain in Thailand five years later.

Afterward, he became involved with a United Nations initiative that developed an education program to focus on a workplace response to

" ... PEOPLE WITH AIDS WERE SCORNED BY FELLOW EMPLOYEES, FIRED FROM THEIR JOBS ... "

AIDS that dealt with contagion and fitness for duty and that also worked to reduce stigma.

While the basis of the conflict was that casual contact did not transmit HIV, the science was almost impossible to sort out from the public relations issues at the corporate level. Another question dealt with the employer's duty to disclose this information to other employees. As in the healthcare industry, the question of disclosure to others was a flashpoint for years.

As people in the boardroom struggled to develop rational corporate policies, people with AIDS were scorned by fellow employees, fired from their jobs, evicted from their apartments, shunned by their families, forced to close their businesses, and they lost their health insurance and their livelihoods. There was little case law for guidance. That would come later.

In the meantime, I was drafted to serve on the New York State Bar Association's Committee on AIDS and the Law, chaired by Rochester attorney, Ross Lanzafame, Esq. I learned a tremendous amount about the huge challenges facing the legal community. I tried to represent the contagion issues so that they were included in the discussion.

While the legal community was gearing up, the Medical Society of the State of New York (MSSNY) began to address AIDS education and policy for its members. I became chair of MSSNY's Subcommittee on AIDS. The need for HIV education and policy has never gone away, and I've stayed for 27 years.

When the nurse was able to go back to work, many felt she should not return to the

I.C.U. It made no scientific sense to me. I held my ground, beating the drum that there was no risk of HIV transmission to patients; it would *not* be necessary to restrict her patient contact in any way. I referred to the experience from Europe where there had been no transmission by an HIV-positive surgeon to patients during surgical procedures.

At a meeting with various administrative people involved, the consensus was to reassign her to the outpatient clinic. One administration colleague presented the administrative perspective. Nobody doubted the science, she said. The decision to restrict the nurse's activities were administrative and took into account the hysteria of the era. There are times when the institutional need overrides the science, and this was one of them.

As I reflect on this all these years later, I can see the wisdom of what was a rational decision at the time. There was never any discussion of terminating this nurse. While our nurse was reassigned, people in the hospital who knew what happened closed ranks around her. She continued working and was treated with dignity and respect.

My learning curve was getting steeper.

I left that meeting feeling like a failure, my stomach in knots, and I rushed back to the clinic. The waiting room was jammed with patients. Adam, a patient with Kaposi's sarcoma, was there and nodded to me, his once good looks now scarred by those miserable raised purple spots all over his face. I was reminded of why I was doing this insane work.

On my way to find Carol, I stopped to talk to Patty Ross, the office manager, who advised me that my medical students were waiting in my office. She also handed me a stack of phone messages, including one from Bob Loeb, the medical center's public information director, about a TV news interview later in the day. I had forgotten that I had sent the students to the library to read up on Kaposi's sarcoma and that Adam had agreed to be the teaching case that day.

I found Carol and pulled her into her office, a well-organized command center. She listened as I related the outcome of the meeting. In a soft voice, she said, "Don't let it get you down. You have bigger battles to fight and a few patients waiting, doctor. "And don't forget—dinner at my house for the staff tonight at 6 p.m."

I still needed to do that TV interview before I left for the day. Recently, Bob Loeb recalled those days when we made every effort to work with local media and he acted as my "agent." Since time was tight and we avoided having TV cameras in the clinic, he set up the camera crew in the hallway between the clinic and my office. When I finished in clinic, I met the reporter in the hallway, did the interview and then headed to Carol's house.

When I arrived at Carol's that evening, a glass of Chablis was waiting.

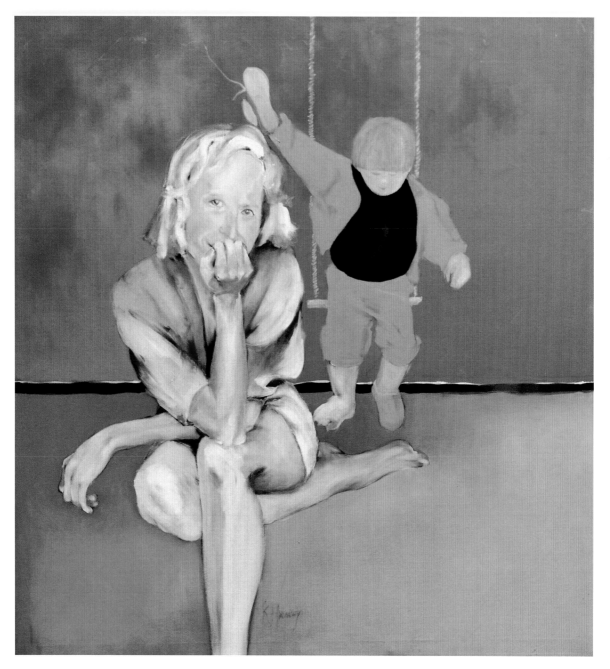

▸ *Mother and Child,* Kathleen Hanney, 1989. A gift of the artist on the opening of Community Health Network, this work speaks to the important roles of mothers early in the epidemic.

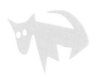

8 | THE NEIGHBORHOOD PAPERBOY: HIS LAST DAY

He was the neighborhood paperboy. His mother and I sat at his bedside after he died. I told her I grew up in the neighborhood and had visited her house many times when a friend from high school lived there.

At first, I saw my patient in the office. His mother would come with him to his appointments. She would say, "I want to make sure he really gets here." My young patient had dropped out of college and returned home when he got sick. Of course, his mother's wisdom prevailed.

He had some trouble with drugs and was a handful. But he and his mother kept his appointments, he took his medicine, and he did well for a long time. When he started to decline, I began to make house calls. He lived in the house of a high school friend in the neighborhood where I grew up. I would stop and have lunch with my mother then walk to his house to check him out. I had to remind myself to enter through the front door when I made these house calls. In my high school days, we always went in and out through the back door.

His mom was always gracious, offering me something to eat or drink. She looked tired, though. One day she said to me, "I know he's going to die. We want to keep him at home so he can die here." Her anguish was palpable. We hugged, and I told her that we would keep him at home.

It was always difficult for me to face the reality of impending death. The experience of

"SHE LOOKED AT HIM AND SOBBED, AND THEN BENT OVER HIM AND KISSED HIS FOREHEAD."

most of my patients dying before their parents was upside down. It wasn't supposed to happen that way. What do you say to a mother whose 26-year-old is going to die? What do you say to any mother whose kid is about to die at any age? It gave me a sick feeling in the pit of my stomach. I wanted to find a way to keep him alive, and I couldn't.

In the early years of the Community Health Network, we had two agencies working on-site coordinating home care. So, the visiting nurse started going to the house to check on him. Several months later, when it looked like he was close to the end and was in the home hospice program, I made another house call. I followed my routine and walked to his house from my mother's.

Their house was on a corner. As I approached, I could see the swimming pool in the yard. It was the middle of a hot summer, and the pool was still covered. I assumed that, because of the demands of their son's illness, his parents never got around to opening the pool.

His mother, very tired and sad looking, greeted me at the door and let me in. He was lying on a hospital bed in the living room. The window was open, and there was a breeze that caught the curtains in the window next to his bed. His pills and a glass of water were on a tray next to the bed. She said, "He's had a fever this morning. I just gave him a sponge bath to cool him down."

I accepted her offer of a glass of ice water and sat in the chair next to the bed. In contrast to so many of my patients, he hadn't lost a lot of weight. There was very little of the typical "AIDS wasting." He looked almost healthy.

He was breathing irregularly. When I put my hand on his arm, he was cold, so I knew that he was close to the end. As is my habit, even when patients are unconscious, I talked to him. As I sat with him, talking about nothing in particular, I could hear his mother putting ice into the glass, so she wasn't gone very long.

While I was talking, he opened his eyes, took a deep breath, sighed, and stopped breathing. He was dead at the age of 26. As I stood up and checked his pulse, I looked out the window at the covered swimming pool. Visions of my high school buddies jumping off the diving board went through my mind. I looked at my patient's face. His eyes were still open. Unlike in the movies, real patients who die with their eyes open do not close them when they take their last breath. I positioned his eyelids over his eyes. He looked like he was asleep.

When his mother came back into the room with the ice water, I put my arm on her shoulder and led her to the bed. She looked at him and sobbed and then bent over him and kissed his forehead. We locked eyes as she said, "I'm glad you were here. Thank you for all you've done for him." Quickly, she composed herself and said, "He never saw me cry in all this time."

She excused herself to call her husband at work to tell him that their son had died. I felt like an eavesdropper and tried to tune out their conversation. She returned and said her husband was on his way home.

For the next half hour or so, until her husband arrived, we sat next to the bed. She held her son's hand as she talked about him as a child—playful, energetic, lovable, how much he enjoyed their pool, that he was the neighborhood paperboy in high school. I told her how much I enjoyed her son's high spirits. Then I told her of my experiences in her house when my friend lived there and that my mother still lived in the house where I grew up, something I had never mentioned before. As we talked, we discovered that her son had been my mother's paperboy. Neither of us had any idea of the depth of our neighborhood connection.

Her husband arrived, and I repeated my recollection of their son as courageous and told him that they were good parents to take care of him until the end. As I was getting ready to leave, I asked her what I asked many families in that era, as uncomfortable as it was. I asked her if I could have his unused AZT. She said what every other mother had said to me in that same situation, "Yes, if it will help someone else." She put pill bottles in a bag, we hugged, and I left.

On the walk back to my mother's house, I thought about what had just happened. I had added another dimension to my old dictum that said your patients are your friends and your friends are your patients. My patients were also my neighbors.

I decided that I should talk more to families about the courage of their children, and that I should thank them for their part in taking care of my patients, their loved ones. After that, I made it a point to share an anecdote or comment about my experience with the patient, even the most difficult ones. I hoped that hearing something good about their child might lighten a mother's burden.

It was still early in the epidemic, and I often avoided going to wakes and funerals. I was the AIDS doctor. What was I supposed to say? "I'm sorry your son/daughter/husband/ wife died before their time? We tried, but it didn't work? They're in a better place? I was without words.

That day, I resolved to get over my bad stomach; I would go to memorial services and wakes. It would be more human to share in a family's grief rather than beating myself up for having failed, and it might provide some closure for all of us. Attending wakes and saying something good about the patient might make me more three-dimensional and less like a talking head.

When I arrived back at my mother's house, we sat at the kitchen table. Here was my own mother, my tiny sainted mother. She was calmly working her cooking artistry in the kitchen as she had for the past 40 years. My father had died two years earlier, and she was cooking for my youngest brother who was still at home. As I watched her, I thought of my patient's mother who cared for her son during his illness—giving him a bath on his last day. At least I had spared my own mother that agony.

I watched her as she worked, her spare rosary beads in her apron pocket, doing what she did so well—taking care of her family. Out of the blue, I said to her that she did a lot for us as a family, and I thanked her for it.

She didn't miss a beat. Smiling, she looked up at me and repeated what she had said a thousand times while we were growing up, "That's because I'm your mother."

As I was preparing to leave, she pulled an envelope out of her apron pocket and gave me a check—her monthly donation to the clinic. "I hope this will help your patients," she said.

I was emotionally drained by the day's experiences with these two mothers and the love they shared for their children.

I kissed my mother goodbye and headed home.

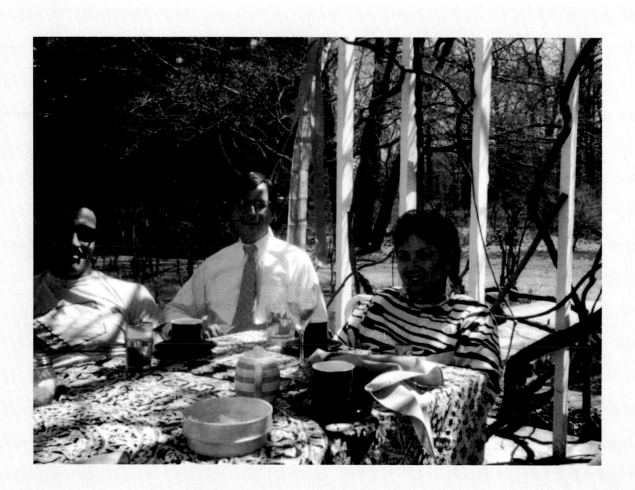

▸ Easter Sunday, 1987. Left to right: Drs. Steve Scheibel, Bill Valenti and Ann Zettelmaier Griepp.

9 | ABOVE THE BUG LINE WITH ANN ZETTELMAIER GRIEPP, M.D.

The early days of AIDS brought people together in different ways. Many of those early professional relationships resulted in lifelong friendships.

—Ann Zettelmaier Griepp, M.D.

We bonded soon after we met. On many nights, we would sit on my upstairs balcony late into the night. My neighbor, who had spent many nights up there chatting with the previous owner of my house, reminded me that the balcony was above the bug line and free of mosquitoes. Ann and I would adjourn from downstairs when the mosquitoes arrived and seek refuge upstairs, drinking coffee and rocking in the hammock. We chatted about the events of the day and the patients who had died, telling anecdotes about them, trying to capture their essence in a positive way. We talked often about writing a book about our experiences and laughed about using *Above the Bug Line* as the title.

The term "above the bug line" became our code for safety or isolation from the wear and tear all of us faced on a daily basis. Everything was OK above the bug line. Down below—not so much. HIV was in our face below the bug line, just like the mosquitoes.

When Ann and I talked about these sessions recently, she recited the names of 20 patients easily. As she said their names, I could see each of their faces. They were not "just patients," Ann said. "I walked closely to death with them, helping them to have joy and resilience, to repair relationships, and to have a death they wanted."

First, the story of how we met. I mentioned to the chief of psychiatry once how badly we needed a psychiatrist in the clinic. He said he had someone in mind. "She's family medicine-trained and one of our best residents."

A few days later, Dr. Ann Zettelmaier appeared in my office. Bright and enthusiastic, she had an engaging personality and a lively sense of humor. I looked at her sitting in the chair across from my desk with that big smile, her right foot carefully tucked under her and her left foot swinging as we talked. I thought to myself, "He sent me a kid. She's so young."

Ann recalled the meeting. "My psychiatry chief believed that AIDS was a place where medicine, neuroscience, and psychotherapy all coalesced. He told me about the AIDS program, and off to the clinic I went. The clinic, all white coats and a waiting room full of patients, was a totally different vibe than the department of psychiatry. In came Bill Valenti, the prototype of what I had come to describe as the 'URMC look': blue button-down collar shirt, tie, khakis, and a white lab coat. He was gracious, pleasant, and multitasking—signing notes or reports."

We set up a plan for Ann to be in the clinic on certain days of the week. Patients who needed therapy could be walked right over to meet her. That was integrated behavioral health in 1986—at least, that's what we would call it now. Or one-stop shopping, as we called it later.

Very quickly, she had a full caseload and became the AIDS psychiatrist. One of our most memorable cases was "the patient with the $200 lunch."

A few months after Ann and I met, I had a phone call about a patient. While phone calls about patients were a daily occurrence, this call was different. The call would highlight Ann's skill as both a family medicine physician and neuropsychiatrist, and it would cement the two of us together.

The manager of The Top of the Plaza restaurant in the old Midtown Plaza, a popular restaurant with a view of the city, was on the phone. One of our patients spent the afternoon having a fine lunch with wine. His bill was more than $200, and he had no money to pay for it. When they found my card in his wallet, he told them to call me.

I was more concerned about the patient's sudden unpredictable behavior than the unpaid food bill, so I instructed the manager to send the patient to the emergency department. The story made no sense, at least at the time. I had seen the patient in the office recently, and he seemed fine. A food and wine *aficionado,* he had returned to Rochester recently from Los Angeles and had been seeing Ann for depression.

Ann and I saw the patient together. I remember us standing at the foot of the patient's bed, watching him, and then looking at each other. He was totally incoherent, mumbling to himself, and laughing. I left to see other patients, and she stayed behind. When I returned, Ann, the emerging neuropsychiatrist, said, "I think we have our first case of AIDS dementia." With further testing, she was correct. It was another unfortunate first in a long line of firsts. HIV dementia was particularly disabling. Often abrupt in onset, it was especially hard to watch in young people.

Over time, we began to understand AIDS dementia and recognize it earlier. We paid more attention to patients who were just a little bit "forgetful." The best treatment at the time was high-dose AZT, since it penetrated the brain. The hope was that the drug might slow HIV brain damage and the patient would improve.

This patient did not improve, and I met with his family to discuss his grim prognosis. They cared for him at home for the rest of his life.

I thought it ironic that on the last day the patient had any semblance of reality, he found his way to a fine restaurant with a view of the city and had a leisurely lunch with some good wine.

Our passion and energy exhausts me when I think about it. The days started early and ended late. Ann recalled the relentless pace: "Start the day with a grand rounds presentation, see patients in the hospital, do an interview with a medical reporter, and have a brown-bag mentoring lunch with residents or therapists starting to treat HIV patients. In the afternoon, attend a meeting about a grant submission, then help set up for a fundraiser, and show up later, dressed to the nines, to welcome attendees. Bigger cities had multiple people playing these roles. In Rochester, a small group 'did it all.' "

Among her many accomplishments was forming a mental health team that grew out of her brown-bag teaching rounds. She also fought to overcome stigma and misinformation. People would often discuss the "innocent victims" of HIV, such as children and people with hemophilia, versus gay men and injection drug users. The harsh judgment in the face of such suffering for bright engaging people and their families was daunting. "It was difficult for me to handle the moral judgment. It made me so angry, and yet my role was to help educate and heal," she said.

As a straight single woman, Ann felt like she was in uncharted waters. Many other friends and family did not understand why she worked with these "dangerous" or "deviant" patients. In this politically charged era, she became the voice of reason, challenging more senior colleagues who espoused sexual reorientation therapy to return a patient to a "heterosexual lifestyle." For a number of years, other psychiatrists and therapists were largely happy to leave the care of these patients to her or to the clinic.

Fortunately, Ann and her chief of psychiatry were aligned, and she pushed ahead and had a remarkable residency experience as the AIDS psychiatrist. In psychiatry, she was part of a world that didn't yet understand and needed help understanding. She said, "Pretty much all I ever did was give lectures, treat patients, hang out with other HIV caregivers, explain the disease and its treatments, write grants, and ask for donations for groups like AIDS Rochester."

Ann and I pulled some "all-nighters" too. Pretending to be Lois Lane and Jimmy Olsen of *Superman* fame, we wrote a major grant for AIDS education on my home Apple II computer with a 6-inch screen. We met the deadline, and the grant was funded.

Despite the pace, we had some notable experiences learning about the disease and its global impact. In 1985, Dr. Robert Gallo came to the medical center to give a lecture on AIDS. Gallo, known for making the connection between the human immunodeficiency virus and AIDS, was the man of the moment. Ann and I were asked to meet him for breakfast during his visit.

Gallo seemed bigger than life to us, so we expected a huge ego and a short meeting. Instead, he was charming, and he was interested in what we were doing and how we were treating patients. We talked for two hours and had a memorable moment in the timeline that would only get more complex as we went on.

In 1988, in the thick of the chaos, Ann and I traveled together to the International AIDS Conference in Stockholm. That year, a group of AIDS advocates dismantled the AZT display booth in the meeting's exhibit hall in protest over AZT's high price. Ann and I discussed the advocacy movement at length after that. We decided that AIDS advocates and medical people were

partners in the effort, with all of us pulling in the same direction to get ahead of the epidemic.

We spent Easter Sundays together for several years. The guest list for Easter at my house often included: Ann, Steve Scheibel, John Washburn, Wally Miller, Adele Fico, Toni Obermeyer, Dr. Rodney Voisine, Dr. Brad Saget, and an eclectic mix of others. We invented games in the Olympic manner, usually with no purpose other than to laugh. We laughed for ourselves and to decompress from situations that brought us together.

The pace was quick—even mourning the loss of patients. Steve Scheibel recalls having ten patients die in the same week. He said that there wasn't time to mourn because we needed to be at our best for the patients who remained and still needed us. Lisa Brozek echoed his sentiment when she said, "we needed to mourn fast and get back to work."

The idea of self-care escaped us. Dr. Hannah Solky, our psychiatrist colleague, constantly reminded us of the importance of self-care. Ann noted that there was no time to slow down. We

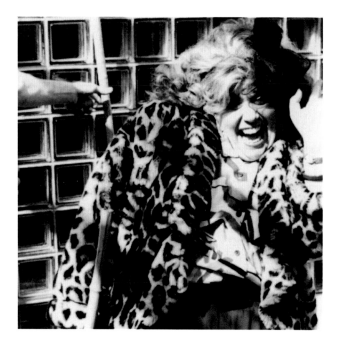

▸ Easter hijinks. Adele Fico, friend and fundraiser, in blond wig and leopard coat, a gift of Dr. John Washburn.

felt we had done the job of self-care if we attended Hannah's weekly support group.

All these years later, Ann said, "Our choices of coping were not always the most adaptive. Pushing boundaries, partying hard, becoming political, and being too focused and intense did not always serve our own personal relationships well." Somehow, our group effort helped us survive. Sadly, a number of notable careers in other cities ended due to drug use, risky sexual behavior, pushing boundaries with patients, or just needing to get out of AIDS care completely.

Ann had her own schedule of AIDS education and service. As a woman of faith, she felt that it was "important to bear witness to the suffering and to understand the value of each patient." She and one of our early patients bonded and often went out together on community speaking engagements. This young man with AIDS wanted to be useful to the effort before he died, and they became regulars at community events, educational programs, and in media interviews. When he died, she spoke at his memorial service.

She recalls the closeness and friendships of those early days in Rochester. The roles and boundaries of our work were constantly blurring. She echoed my experience of patients as friends and friends as patients. "It was a fact of life for me," she remembers.

Ann said it this way, "We bonded through loss which only strengthened our resolve. We played often and hard, surrounding ourselves with art, beauty, and humor as a defense to the pain we saw daily. Our Sunday games with our volleyball teams, 'The Lizards' and 'The Snakes,' were simply awful.

"We had to believe in life and hope to help those who were losing hope. Bill was much better than I at always returning the conversation to research, treatment advances, and hope. As a good physician, Bill saw the main focus as medical care. He wanted to beat AIDS."

One day we were chatting, and Ann said, "I'd like to get married at your house." I told her she would need a good man, a warm day, and a tent. In 1990, she got all three, and she and Jim Griepp were married at my house. She said, "Any man I dated would have to be able to swim in this world. It was not always easy on them. My husband was able to traverse these waters but not without some challenging moments." At times, she longed for a world of children, Little League, and church instead of illness, death, and controversy.

As more people joined the fight and with her treatment team in place, she was eventually able to create the space to have a husband and family life that did not revolve around HIV. We remained connected, and, later, I became the godfather to their son. Our families socialized, and the Griepp family was a part of our family Christmas celebrations for the next 25 years.

She went on, "I did not know then that Bill would become one of my dearest friends in Rochester. I had lived in Michigan and Los Angeles prior to coming to Rochester for my residency. I had experienced Rochester as a bit conservative and aloof. This all changed with the beginning of the HIV work. I was warmly embraced by the gay community—trusted, accepted, and included."

As the AIDS psychiatrist, Ann dispensed professional and personal advice during that era and has been a loyal confidante. She helped keep us all sane during a time of chaos, she helped thousands of patients, and she saved countless lives in the course of her AIDS work.

What remains for us? "Two thoughts," she said. "One is for my daughter to get married at Bill's house and the other is to see the end of AIDS before we finish our careers."

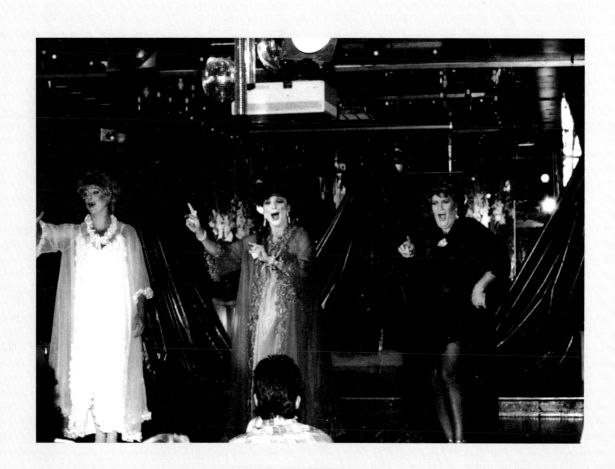

▸ Left to right: Dick Easton, Bill Valenti, and Dan Meyers singing "Dreamgirls," December 1989. Hair stylings by Angelo D'Amico.

10 | ANYTHING FOR THE CAUSE

I learned quickly that fundraising and asking people for money went with the territory. Fundraising events should not only be financially successful, they should help galvanize the community around the AIDS crisis.

Our fundraising efforts were often reported in the media. I enjoyed these activities because they put a lighter tone on the darker events that were unfolding in the clinic.

At the same time, we became fair game for media critics who evaluated our performances more on our artistic abilities and less on science.

Singing. In 1989, we wowed audiences as a trio called "The Mothers." Dick Easton, Dan Meyers, and I wore matching *peignoirs* in white, black and red, respectively. We reprised a number that we had performed four years earlier at a friend's 40th birthday party. We sang "Dreamgirls" as the mothers of three younger drag performers, also on stage that night. Of course, the audience loved it, and we raised several thousand dollars.

Ballet. A year later, on the heels of this success, I approached my next role a bit overconfidently. A local dance impresario asked us to perform in his annual Christmas performance of *The Nutcracker* as a CHN fundraiser. We made our debut on the Eastman Theatre stage.

The "Arabian Dance" had been billed as the most sensual and erotic dance in all of ballet. Steve Scheibel was a magnificent shirtless, well-oiled Arabian with arms crossed and wearing a loin cloth, courtesy of the show's enthusiastic costume designer.

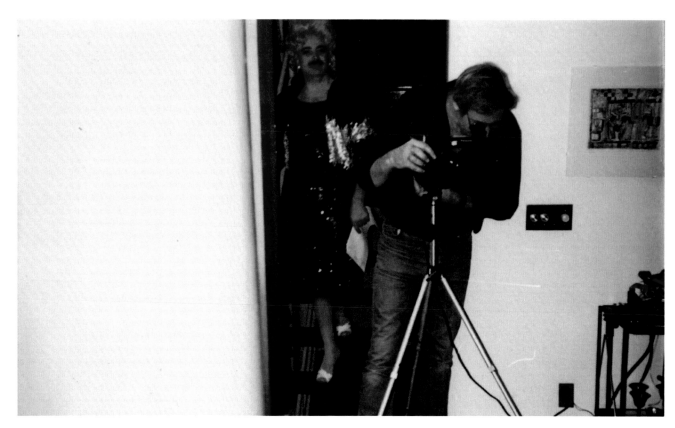

▶ Wally Miller was the videographer for our home movie. The mysterious blond woman on the stairway behind him makes her entrance with script in hand. Adele Fico and Ann Zettelmaier Griepp wrote the script and lyrics.

I was cast as the character Mother Gigogne (Mother Ginger) and wore a gigantic, 10-foot-in-diameter hoop skirt. I stood on 3-foot wooden stilts, the size of small tree stumps, that were strapped to my legs up to my thighs. A 40-pound harness to support the voluminous red skirt and Mother's tall, floppy hat completed the costume. Fully dressed, this gigantic thespian was almost 10 feet off the floor.

"Places, everyone," shouted the director, who instructed me to give an oversized wave over my head as I entered stage left so that the audience in the back rows could appreciate the wonder of it all. I was reminded that Mother Gigogne was a humorous, silly character and that I should wave my arms and laugh as the children danced in front of me. I winced. I should have backed out sooner. It was too late now.

I shuffled onto the stage sideways, being careful not to step on one of the dozen 5-year-old "ginger babies" crawling and giggling beneath my skirt. One false move, and I would be on the floor, children would be crushed, and the show would be over. I was feeling the pressure.

When I reached center stage, the kids popped out from under the skirt and did their dance. Instead of being silly and amusing while the kids danced, I stood there, frozen, and fearful that I would tip over. Their dance finished, and the kids scurried back under Mother's skirt for the exit.

I completed this delicate balancing act without breaking my legs or stepping on a kid. I exited stage right, and it was over.

The local paper's dance critic wrote about the event the next morning in a biting critique in which he called the show "a mixed dose of medicine," and referred to us as "moonlighting MDs." He went on: "Valenti had no idea what to do with the mugging role of 'Mother Gigogne,' but his friends in the audience whooped it up, ignoring the snappy dancing by the kids who emerged from under Mother G's enormous skirts." Obviously, the critic failed to appreciate my gymnastic skills.

Film. Our little gang made a movie in 1989. A group of us gathered at my house during the Christmas holidays. After dinner, we filmed a parody of a popular holiday special of the era, *An Andy Williams Christmas Special*. My dinner guests and I had the speaking and singing parts.

After we viewed this outrageous, irreverent video, we realized that none of us could ever run for public office or be a Supreme Court justice. So we all agreed not to show the movie to others and to keep it to ourselves.

Fast forward to April 1995. Helping People with AIDS roasted me in a fundraiser with the usual barbs flying. The headline in the *Democrat and Chronicle* the next morning, April 2, 1995: "Valenti Roasted in HPA Fundraiser."

The guests all wore one-piece masks with dark glasses and big noses. Very funny so far. The reporter in attendance wrote about Dan Meyers' safe sex "demonstration" that ended with him dressed completely in plastic. A hit!

My mood changed when Toni Obermeyer followed me to the microphone. The lights went down, and on comes the 1989 movie we had pledged to keep in the archives.

The morning paper described it this way: "Toni Obermeyer, former outreach worker at AIDS Rochester who now lives in New York City and is a frequent houseguest of Valenti's, showed her videotape of a singing Marilyn Monroe, portrayed by a lip-synching Valenti in drag."

Toni called the next morning. She asked if I had seen the morning paper.

Bill: "Along with everyone else in town, including my mother who reads the paper front to back every day. Tone, my brother and sister-in-law were in the audience. And, you will remember that I was Zsa Zsa Gabor in the movie, not Marilyn!"

Toni: "Well, they said it was a roast. Now be a good boy, and call your mother."

And so it was.

A Movie Queen to Play the Scene: Elizabeth Taylor

Elizabeth Taylor was the consummate AIDS fundraiser, raising millions through her own foundation and the American Foundation for AIDS Research (amfAR) that she co-founded with Dr. Michael Gottlieb. She came on the AIDS scene when the matinée idol Rock Hudson came out as a man with AIDS. When Hudson died in October 1985, he was the first high-profile celebrity to die of AIDS. Hudson's death put AIDS on the front pages of newspapers for months afterward. Elizabeth Taylor then became a major force in the battle against AIDS.

By the beginning of 1985, more than 5,500 people had died of AIDS in the U.S.

Except for a few mentions about AIDS at press conferences and in a State of the Union address, the Reagan White House remained silent.

I shook hands with Elizabeth Taylor in 1991 at the International Conference on AIDS in Florence, Italy, where we presented a paper on CHN's Eye Watch program. She made a brief appearance at an amfAR cocktail reception. I arrived early and stood in front of the platform where she would speak to us, so I had a front-row seat.

Elizabeth arrived with several of her handlers. She was stunningly beautiful, as expected. As she took the stage, I noted that, ever so smoothly, she handed her tiny purse to one of the young men escorting her. Great style.

Unscripted, she spoke passionately about our priorities—the need for acceptance of people with AIDS, funding needs, research priorities, and reducing stigma. She drove the point home by saying that "PEOPLE ARE DYING!" She said those words with the same passion as she confronted Katherine Hepburn in *Suddenly, Last Summer* in 1959. The young man next to me was wiping back tears as she spoke. It was gripping.

She closed by thanking us for the work that we did. In 10 minutes, she made a huge impact and validated the work we were doing.

When she finished, I was close enough to rush the stage and talk to her. I don't remember what I said. She looked up at me, smiled, and said thank you. Then her handlers rushed her away, and it was over. Truly memorable!

I wrote a check to amfAR when I returned to the U.S.

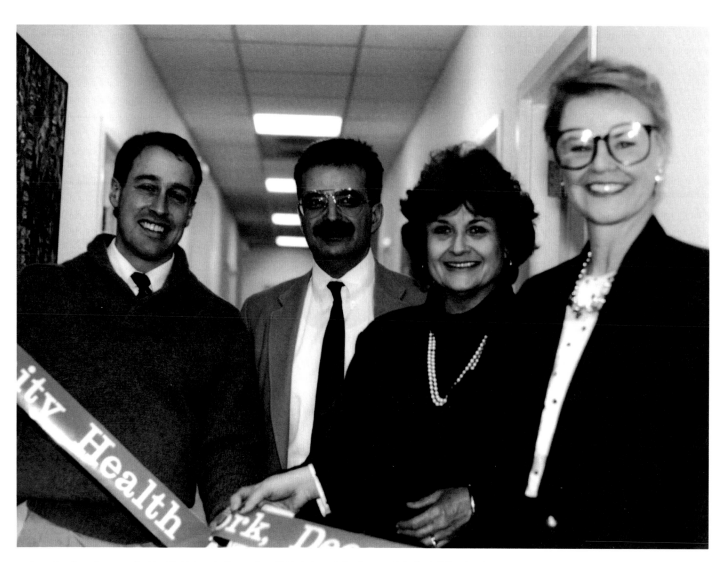

▸ Opening Day, Community Health Network, December 1989. Left to right: Steven Scheibel, Bill Valenti, U.S. Representative Louise Slaughter, and Carol Williams.

11 | COMMUNITY HEALTH NETWORK: A TEAM EFFORT

We thought that if we did this right, we would create a health organization that would outlast any of us. At the same time, we were creating a corporate culture that would set the stage for the organization long-term.

My last day at The Strong Memorial clinic was December 21, 1988. The program was now in the capable hands of Dr. Amy Portmore who had joined the program several years earlier. Dr. Michael Keefer became clinic director in 1990. Mike is still fighting the fight today. Among his many accomplishments, he has gone on to guide our HIV vaccine research efforts locally and on the global stage.

Armed with my university training that included the art and science of medicine and the art of the sound bite, I was now a free agent; an unemployed free agent. Linda Bennett, one of our secretaries in the Infectious Diseases Unit, joined us soon afterward as CHN's office manager and worked from my home office until we opened. One day, I told her that I was unsure about being unemployed. She smiled and said, "Then call yourself 'physician-at-large,'" a title I would use from time to time over the years. I continued with the CHN planning. To pay the mortgage, I went on the road and gave lectures for the few HIV drug manufacturers at the time.

The engagements were always stimulating, kept me current, and allowed me to see the current state of HIV care in the U.S. and around the world. It appeared that if CHN succeeded, we would be unique as a community-based program since most HIV care at the time was done in hospitals.

Along the way, I met many others who were also fighting the fight. My AIDS Institute committee work took me regularly to New York City, the epicenter of the epidemic. The AIDS Institute made a strong commitment to include community people, patients, and advocates in their work. It became clear to me that the medical community alone would not win this battle. Instead, the advocacy movement would be equal partners in the fight.

The intensity of the New York City experience helped give some context to what I was doing. While we were overwhelmed in Rochester, the sheer volume of patients in New York City was an entirely different dynamic in terms of connecting people to medical care and services.

Dr. Linda Laubenstein was an early AIDS warrior. Based at New York University, she and her collaborators published the first paper describing the relationship between Kaposi's sarcoma (KS) and AIDS in 1982. I met her at a committee meeting. A tiny woman in a wheelchair, I recognized her immediately. She was a polio survivor, and I knew her story from an article in *The New York Times* that described her role as an AIDS doctor and researcher. The photo accompanying the article showed her making a house call in her wheelchair and being carried up the stairs of a New York City walk-up by two men. The image was seared in my brain as was the article's description of her making house calls using public buses. I went over to her and introduced myself. I told her of my experiences and lack of success with KS in Rochester and talked to her about a troubling case I had. She said, "Call me anytime." And I did.

She died at the age of 45 in 1992. She lives on as the inspiration for the character Dr. Emma Booker in Larry Kramer's play *The Normal Heart* about the early days of the AIDS epidemic.

Later, the AIDS Institute would name their Clinical Excellence Award after her. I received the award in 2013, a humbling experience for me on so many levels.

The Clinic

We called CHN "the clinic" from day one. We thought that the term stated very clearly that we were about healthcare. We avoided the term "the practice," preferring to align ourselves with the Mayo Clinic image or the more European style of a destination for healthcare. We wanted it to be a bastion of civility amidst the chaos.

Community Health Network was a gamble. My medical school roommate and lifelong friend Dr. Bruce Hinrichs said in a letter of endorsement that he wrote for me that my "career path change, while risky, was necessary for the time." As I think back, I am still in awe of the people who were willing to take the risk with us and sign on to an idea that was a work in progress. Obviously, the AIDS crisis drove people to get involved. In retrospect, CHN was a community collaboration; I was merely the catalyst.

Steve Scheibel, Carol Williams, and Sidney Metzger interrupted careers and secure positions at the University of Rochester to sign on. Others invested money and time in an organization that was yet to be created.

The New York State legislature created the AIDS Institute by statute in 1985. Since 1987, another AIDS warrior, Dr. Nick Rango, was heading this new arm of the state health department. I met Nick at various committee meetings, and he was no-nonsense, passionate, and visionary. One day in early 1989, Steve and I went to New York to explain our idea to Nick and one of his associates. In those days, the AIDS Institute consisted of a few dark rooms at the end of a long hallway at 100 Center Street. More to the point, they were all business. They thought the clinic was a great idea but an "expensive model" because of the overhead, salaries, and cash flow with billing. Nick made a financial commitment on the spot to get us started.

We explained the concept. In addition to a clinic that would provide primary and specialty HIV care, there would also be an AIDS Rochester satellite office, a substance-abuse program, two home-care agencies, a patient lab, and a pharmacy on one site. The agencies would rent space from us to help offset the costs. Rango was right about it being expensive. Scheibel and I took a salary of $1,000 a month for the first year. We needed to pay our staff.

About six months after we opened, I was in New York for a meeting, and Nick invited me to

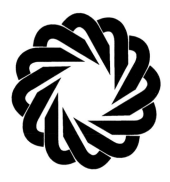

▶ The mandala, CHN's logo, signifies spirituality, healing, enlightenment, compassion, and wholeness.

dinner at his Greenwich Village apartment. While his mother served us lasagna and garlic bread, I briefed him on our progress. He reminded me again that CHN was the first of its kind in the state and that Valenti and Scheibel were on the hook for all operating costs. People in the health department "were watching" to see if our model worked so that it might be rolled out elsewhere, so he was on the hook also. I told him that I had

$65,000 from my own shrinking bank account in the project, and I promised him we wouldn't fail.

Still, we had our detractors who thought we would fail or, worse yet, questioned the need for a community-based AIDS clinic at all. We pushed ahead. Steve Scheibel said, "We can't fail; the work is too important."

The work we did to get this far was grueling and unrelenting. At the same time, doors opened for us. Individuals, fundraising groups, foundations, businesses and the government were generous and interested in doing something about AIDS. Added together, the initial contributions—dollars and in-kind—from the Rochester community at all levels totaled more than a million dollars. In truth, those contributions were immeasurable.

Our early "leap of faith" investors were Wegmans; Gannett Foundation; Fred and Floy Willmott Foundation; Rochester Primary Care Network; United Way; The Daisy Marquis Jones Foundation; Rochester Community Individual Practice Association, the physician arm of the local Blue Choice HMO; St. Mary's Hospital Foundation; Blue Cross/Blue Shield of the Rochester Area; Preferred Care; Max Adler

Foundation; Davenport-Hatch Foundation; a friend and local philanthropist Dick Brush; and my own mother, Rose Valenti. A year later, we received a vote of confidence and a donation from the Ames-Amzalak Trust through the Rochester Area Foundation as the most innovative nonprofit project of 1989.

When I was given the Rochester evening paper's endorsement as their "Person of the Year" for 1989, I made it clear that I didn't do any of this by myself. Whatever I have accomplished has been done with the help of thousands of people, many of whom are mentioned in this book.

In 1988, Mary Ellen Burris was Director of Consumer Affairs at Wegmans. We first met when we both served on the county Board of Health in the mid-1980s. From the moment we met, we liked each other. She became an ally and has remained so to this day. In a series of meetings over a year, we crafted a corporate culture and style for the yet-to-be-created organization that would be welcoming and, most of all, provide a "one-stop-shopping" experience for patients.

Fortunately, we followed Pearl Ruben's advice and would become a not-for-profit. Pearl, then executive director of The Daisy Marquis Jones Foundation, said our idea for an AIDS clinic would only work as a nonprofit, not a "private practice." I called Susan Robfogel, a friend who had been involved in the CHN idea from the beginning. She was overseeing the work for us to become a legal entity. Recently, we recalled a 1988 dinner at my house with Steve Scheibel. She and her husband, Nick, agreed to help us in any way they could. Susan put me in contact with Carolyn Kent, an associate at her firm, now Nixon Peabody, to help with our designation as a 501c3 charity under the IRS code. Under Carolyn's direction, we were designated in record time, and Carolyn became a member of our first board, later serving as board president.

By now, we had adopted the Scheibel theme of "taking the path of least resistance." He describes this as "water streaming down the side of a mountain" in the foreword to this book. In other words, if someone or some organization could not or chose not to be involved, we would move on and work with those who were interested. We went around town to meet with various people and present the idea of an AIDS clinic to see if they could help in some way. First, we would ask for money. Steve insisted that beggars shouldn't be choosers. If people couldn't donate funds, we'd ask if they could assign personnel to assist. If that wasn't possible, "we'd ask to use their fax machine." It worked.

We needed a name for this "entity." A friend who worked in public relations locally put together a volunteer communications/PR group. These seasoned PR people conducted focus groups, did surveys, and offered advice. We learned that people wanted a discreet, private entrance and didn't want AIDS in the name.

After considering hundreds of options, the name Community Health Network won out. The space we had rented was on the lower level of 758 South Avenue with an entrance off the back parking lot, so it checked all the boxes. Also, there was never a sign over the door—there was only a sign in front that listed us as "CHN" along with other building tenants.

After lengthy discussions, we settled on a logo suggested by Lynette Loomis, one of our PR advisors. We chose the mandala that signifies spirituality, healing, enlightenment, compassion, and wholeness. The mandala had meaning for the chaos going on around us. We used it for many years.

As a charitable organization, we needed a New York State license to operate. In his get-it-done style, Nick Rango reminded us constantly, "You need an Article 28," which was a New York State Health Department operating certificate under Article 28 of the Public Health Law. The state health department would try to truncate the usual two-year approval process.

The Turning Point

One day in early 1989, we found ourselves at the offices of Rochester Blue Cross/Blue Shield. Tony Amado was senior vice-president of home care and was active in community AIDS organizations. Tony and his wife were strong allies and supporters of the effort, and he liked our idea. One night over dinner at their house, he said that Howard Berman, the Blues CEO, might be interested in our idea and offered to set up a meeting. Up until then, our concept was embraced enthusiastically but didn't have legs.

Steve and I presented the idea to their senior management team, and they liked it—but not before Howard Berman gave me a quick lesson in brevity. I opened the presentation with a long-winded discussion of the need for an AIDS clinic. He stopped me as I was doing a grand rounds-like discussion and asked me with a smile, "What is it that you want?" I responded, "Your resources. The health department said we needed something called an Article 28 license." He looked at me and said, "I have one of those." We were now on track. The result was that this yet-to-be-born entity would become a satellite

> ## "I TOLD HOWARD BERMAN THAT THE HEALTH DEPARTMENT SAID WE NEEDED AN ARTICLE 28 LICENSE. HE LOOKED AT ME AND SAID, 'I HAVE ONE OF THOSE.'"

clinic of the Blues' Genesee Valley Group Health, now known as Lifetime Health. Berman took our idea and brought it to life.

That day, Berman introduced Margaret "Peggy" Montaglione, now Clark, then vice- president of Group Health. He pulled her out of a meeting, and we chatted in the doorway. Berman explained his idea to Peggy, and, smiling, she agreed enthusiastically. The rest, as they say, is history. We were on our way. Scheibel and I went back to my house that evening, cooked dinner, and celebrated with a bottle of Chianti.

During our collaboration, it became obvious that Peggy Clark had created health centers from the ground up before. She assigned the task of the Article 28 application to her staffer, Christine Bentley. I had known Christine since my infectious diseases fellowship days. Her husband, Dr. David Bentley, was chief of infectious diseases at Monroe Community Hospital and was passionate about infectious diseases in the elderly and chronically ill.

David was another mentor who helped shape my thinking, especially about the value of public health research, so-called "population research." The highlight of my time with David was our publishing collaboration. His attention to detail has stayed with me all these years. One of his mantras was, "Write your first draft of a paper, and then throw it away and start over from the beginning." I have followed his advice many times over the years. At any rate, our second research paper together was published in *The New England Journal of Medicine,* a major achievement for someone with my limited experience as an investigator.

Christine was equally exacting in her role. Our collaboration writing the Article 28 application was a pleasure and a steep learning curve for me. It was obvious she had done this before and could do it in her sleep. The process was fast-paced and involved hundreds of meetings and phone calls. The Group Health satellite clinic designation gave us some breathing room while our own Article 28 licensing application worked its way quickly through the health department.

The Finger Lakes Health Systems Agency (HSA) was a helpful partner—another example of the community pulling together. In this case, the health department required the HSA's blessing for the Article 28 license approval.

The contingency on the HSA sign-off was that we needed expanded clinic hours—either a weekday until 7 p.m. or a Saturday morning. We chose Tuesday evening. For the past 27 years, I have been joined on Tuesday evenings by a team like no other. While I have seen patients on 95 percent of those Tuesday evenings, the multidisciplinary team working with me has done the heavy lifting—keeping the vision alive, providing service to patients who needed evening appointments, and making me look good in the process.

Peggy Clark, Steve Scheibel, and I went to Albany to meet with the health department on Valentine's Day 1990. We wanted to discuss the arrangement with Group Health and check on our own application's progress. They told us we were on track, and we celebrated with chocolate candy in the mall beneath the health department complex. Nick Rango, Peggy Clark, Christine Bentley, and Carol Williams all pulled together on this one, and we crossed the finish line. Within a year, we would be fully approved as a New York State Health Department-licensed Article 28 "Diagnostic and Treatment Center."

Later, our accountants, Jerry Archibald and Mario Urso, led us through the development of our "business plan." At the meeting where they introduced the topic of a business plan, I had no idea what they were talking about. It seemed to me that a project with such a noble purpose was enough to carry the day. I soon learned otherwise. We developed the plan, set our rates, and created billing and fee arrangements with insurers and Medicaid. We also created a professional corporation for billing: "Valenti and Scheibel PC."

But, before I get ahead of myself, we did hit a snag before opening: a construction shutdown in April 1989.

While Peggy Clark was overseeing the birth of a state-licensed clinic and Susan Robfogel was leading our incorporation. Many people still remember the combined exam room and office that we used, while the construction of the clinic was taking place downstairs in the former Elk's Club bowling alley. Our secretary, Linda Bennett, was still working out of my home office, and when the office was being used for patients, I made phone calls from my car phone in the parking lot.

Tom Somerville, a local artist and photographer, was our first patient, and he described his experience. He had a 9 a.m. appointment on day one, Thursday, July 6, 1989, when we opened in temporary space. He recalled that Steve Scheibel met him in the parking lot to escort him inside, since the main entrance to the clinic was still under construction.

Temporary turned out to be longer than we thought. The city had stopped construction because of permit problems. At any rate, the day we learned of the shutdown, Carol Williams, Steve Scheibel, and I sat in our one-room office and stared at the floor.

I thought to myself, "What have we gotten ourselves into?" At the same time, I realized that there was no turning back. We would figure this out. A donor had scheduled a cocktail party fundraiser that evening, so we were torn. For no particular reason, we decided that music was in

" ... I REALIZED THAT THERE WAS NO TURNING BACK."

order, and one of us started singing. Next, we were all on our feet as we laughed and danced our version of an Irish jig to decompress, wondering if there was a regulation forbidding dancing in a state-licensed clinic. Then we went to the party and regrouped the next day.

While we waited for the construction stoppage to be resolved, we continued to see patients in our upstairs makeshift clinic. The waiting room was in the hallway. Our patients were tough, loyal, and determined. Once again, we all pulled together.

Once the space was built out, Neal Parisella, a local designer, decorated the space. Neal's idea was that, despite a limited budget, CHN would not look like any other doctor's office. With Group Health's contribution of waiting room and exam room furnishings and a telephone system, Neal put the rest of the place together with a lot of gray Formica, carpeting, and spatter paint. To round out the furnishings, a friend, Shirley King, stepped in. Shirley, a human resources manager at Mobil Chemical in Rochester, offered us a trip to the company's retired furniture warehouse to furnish the conference room, boardroom, and other areas. Best of all, Shirley arranged for delivery.

With Highland Hospital two blocks away from CHN, it made sense to admit patients there. Their welcome was, in a word, extraordinary.

Highland's management team, including Dr. Howard Beckman, then chief of medicine, and John Lee, vice-president, would prove to be strong advocates for us. We learned to rely on Highland for some of the necessities, and they helped willingly. After all these years, John Lee and I still laugh about the day he dropped by to check in on us. I asked him to buy name badges for our growing clinic staff. (I was shameless.) He was happy to help.

St. Mary's Hospital, where we also admitted patients, was another huge booster and was one of the first hospitals in the community to welcome AIDS patients. Of course, it helped having an enlightened Bishop like Matthew Clark who saw the effort as part of their ministry for AIDS patients.

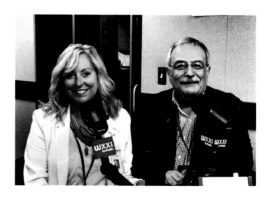

▶ Andrea DeMeo and Bill Valenti promoting Courage, Hope and Innovation.

Once we opened, another benefit of the Highland connection was that its residents rotated through CHN and learned something about AIDS care. Some memorable residents of the era who spent time with us learned about HIV and helped ease the crush of patients. One was the affable, energetic Dr. Charles "Chuck" Cavallaro, currently an emergency medicine physician in Rochester.

Back on track, opening day, Monday, December 4, 1989, finally arrived. It was an exciting day, packed with people and media. Hundreds of supporters were there throughout the day. At the ribbon-cutting, Congresswoman Louise Slaughter summarized the moment. In her remarks, she said, "The work of this clinic will transform AIDS in ways we cannot appreciate today. Along with needed medical care, Community Health Network will give patients comfort and a refuge from this illness. This clinic will provide needed medical care, hope, and, maybe, someday, a cure."

Fast forward to January 2015: On her first day as CEO of Trillium Health, the former CHN, Andrea DeMeo summarized the "past as prologue." I thought my heart stopped as she spoke, "This organization was founded on courage, hope, and innovation."

Twenty-five years apart, Louise and Andrea both nailed it.

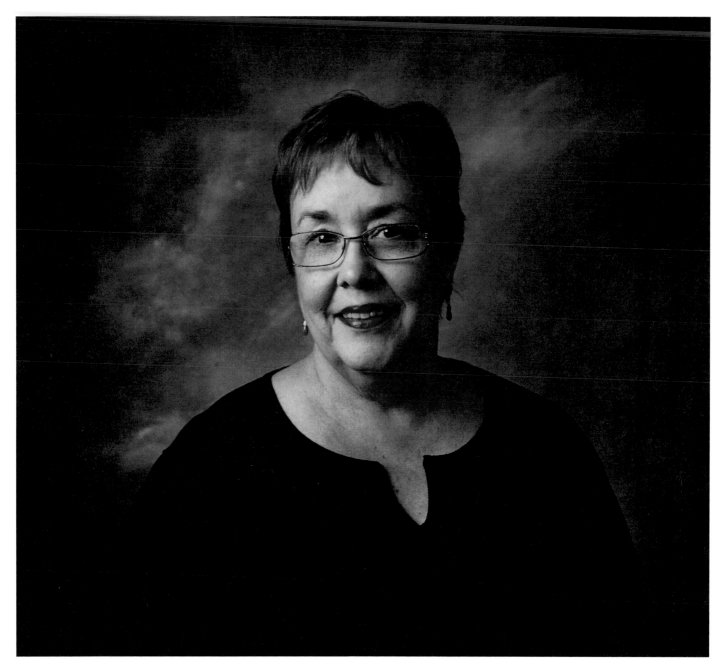

▸ Sidney Wilson Metzger (1936-2014) invented HIV social work in a community-based setting.

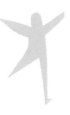

12 | THE SOCIAL WORKER: SIDNEY "SID" METZGER

Sidney Metzger will be remembered for her social activism, for advocating for reproductive rights, and for being a founding member of Community Health Network. When United Way gave us a two-year grant for a social worker's salary, we called Sid and offered her the job. She accepted on the spot.

Sid and I first met on the inpatient units at Strong Memorial when we were starting the HIV program there. She was the social worker on the gynecology service, and one day, she called and asked me for my help.

During the planning phase for the hospital's AIDS center, we all agreed that we would not establish an "AIDS unit." Instead, we went with what proved to be the wiser decision of a "scatter bed" approach in which patients would be admitted to available beds, mostly on the medical service. It worked 99 percent of the time, but there were times when the need exceeded capacity. Sid's call was about a man with AIDS who was admitted to the gynecology floor since it was the last bed in the hospital. The staff was anxious about the situation, so I went to the floor to meet with them. I did an educational session that helped to relieve some of the anxiety.

Sid and I got to know each other better after that. I admired her because she "got it." We could have a conversation and accomplish something. To this day, I like that kind of interaction. When it clicks, it clicks, and that's a beautiful thing. She once sent me a note after she retired that said, "I followed you once, and I'd do it again."

When we opened Community Health Network in 1989, we were swamped with patients. By mid-1990, we had grown from 75 patients to 450. We were desperate for a social worker to help with our patients' complicated situations with housing, insurance, employment, and family issues.

United Way rescued us with a grant for two years' salary for a social worker. We hired Sid, and we were on our way. She asked me before she started her job, "What is it that you want me to do?"

We laughed about this over the years. I said, "I don't know. Social work stuff. You'll figure it out." And she did. Her office was strategically located in the clinic behind the front desk, so she knew everything that happened. I can see her in her office with the blue jar of condoms on her desk. A multitasker like the rest of us, she would be talking on the telephone, writing in a patient's chart, and monitoring the situation in the front office.

There are many stories that capture her essence. One took place sometime after CHN opened in 1989. Sid, Steve Scheibel, our head nurse Carol Williams, and I were at a social event.

We did a brief presentation on AIDS, promoting CHN in the process. After we spoke, a well-dressed woman of a certain age approached us. She looked us all over and said something like, "Well, you two are the doctors." Then she looked at Carol and said, "And you are the nurse." Then she looked at Sid and said, "Just what is it that you do?" Sid replied with a smile, "Everything else!"

The Moms

Mothers played an active role in their children's healthcare in that early era. So many mothers accompanied their children to their appointments. Sid recognized a need and worked to find a way to support all of the mothers we encountered as we began seeing the many once-healthy young men—boys, really—struck down by AIDS. Their moms did not stand by and watch their kids die. Mothers were the "silent" victims, but they needed a collective voice.

Sid organized and led the group that became the Mothers' Support Group, a.k.a. "The Moms," that included Cora Mancuso, Barbara Wickstrom, and Ramona Frank. If it was Monday at 10 a.m., we knew where to find Sid—with "The Moms."

Cora Mancuso's son Fred lost his vision due to cytomegalovirus (CMV) retinitis, a particularly cruel opportunistic infection in those days. In his 30s, he moved back to Rochester and gave up a design career in New York City. He was a smart, witty, handsome devil.

Cora and Fred came to every appointment together. She was also his advocate and his eyes. I can still hear her voice as she led him down the hall. "This way, Freddie. Good morning, doctor." And she always had a smile for everyone, despite her pain. One of my many memories of Fred was his wit. He was blind, but he kept his sense of humor.

Many of "The Moms" stayed connected to the clinic after their children died. Cora Mancuso volunteered at AIDS Rochester. Nancy Zea, whose brother was an early patient, is a Trillium volunteer to this day. Gini Keck, the editor of this book, took care of her son George before he died and later joined our board of directors and helped out in marketing and development.

I'm thankful for Sid and the many moms who sought refuge and support as they tried to forestall the inevitable. These were cruel days for everyone.

When Sid died in 2014, Rich Fowler, a longtime Trillium employee, wrote:

It is with a heavy heart that we share the news of the loss of our dear friend and colleague Sidney Metzger. Sid, as she was known to most, is recognized as one of the founding members of Community Health Network, a legacy agency of Trillium Health.

A career social worker known for her compassion and empathy, Sid's contributions to the HIV/AIDS community are the foundation on which many programs still in existence today were based. A woman of style and grace, she had the ability to make anyone feel welcome and comfortable regardless of circumstance.

We offer our sincerest condolences to the Metzger family and the eclectic circle of friends and colleagues that she welcomed as her extended family.

She did, indeed, have style and grace—and her diplomacy was another strong suit. In addition to healing with her wisdom, Sid was a healer with food.

After joining CHN in early 1990, she invited Strong's infectious diseases clinic staff for lunch at CHN to see the place. I had misgivings about it, but she prevailed. Sid was *very* persuasive that way. I knew she was right once the activity got under way.

Our conference room table was set very elegantly with china and linen—obviously brought from her house on West Brook Road—and the food was all Sid. The two groups chatted like old friends. It was a relief. Not only did she help break the ice, but she also helped set the tone for collaboration between CHN and Strong that needed to happen. It was good for everyone in the end.

That was one of many occasions where Sid, like Carol Williams, persuaded me to look at things through a different lens. I'm glad I did, and I thanked her many times for that.

Her legacy, however, is the work she did with our patients. I honestly believe that Sid was the "inventor" of HIV social work/care management in a community medical setting. It was 1990 after all, and up to that time, most AIDS care was done in hospitals.

Patients still talk about her. I was having a conversation with a long-time patient recently, and Sid's name came up. The patient was going through a rough time, and I was trying to encourage him a bit. During the conversation, I said something about looking at his situation in a different way to help him "move beyond it." He put his head back against the wall, closed his eyes, and said, "You know, Sid Metzger told me the same thing a long time ago. She helped a lot of people, didn't she?"

I agreed. "She was the best."

AIDS on Film

By the time the film *Philadelphia* arrived in 1994, more than 800 cases of AIDS had been reported in Rochester, and several thousand people were estimated to be HIV-positive. In August of that year, I attended the 10th International AIDS Conference in Yokohama, Japan. The good news was that combinations of HIV drugs were starting to work, and one report said that this treatment made it possible to keep HIV patients healthy and alive. "HIV doesn't need to be a death sentence," declared one researcher. At that point, more than 400,000 cases of AIDS had been reported in the U.S. with more than 2.5 million reported in Asia.

The local newspaper invited our clinic group to a pre-screening of Jonathan Demme's film at The Little Theatre in February 1994. This was the first effort of a Hollywood studio to discuss AIDS, homosexuality, and homophobia. In his Academy Award-winning performance as best actor, Tom Hanks played Andrew Beckett, a Philadelphia lawyer who had been fired by his firm when it was learned that he had AIDS. The story was gut-wrenching and vivid. We sat there, riveted, watching Hanks slowly die of AIDS.

Hanks' character is an opera buff, and the classical music in the film is extraordinary. Sid, an opera buff in her own right, was sitting next to me. As we listened and wiped the tears from our eyes, she whispered to me that the mournful arias we were hearing were sung by the legendary diva, Maria Callas, one of my father's favorites. Callas' two arias, translated from the Italian,

" ... WATCHING IT ON THE SCREEN WAS STILL RAW."

were "Well? I Shall Go Far Away" and "The Dead Mother." In the haunting scene where Callas sings "The Dead Mother" in Italian, Hanks moves about the room attached to an IV pole, passionately lip synching and translating the aria for Washington. I watched this scene again recently and was once more reduced to tears.

I was wiped out by this viewing experience. It had been 13 years since the first reports of AIDS, and watching it on the screen was still raw. It was like going to work. I tried to imagine how many opera buffs with AIDS spent their last days finding solace in the voice of Maria Callas. Sid, the healer and mind-reader, rubbed my elbow and whispered, "Think of how comforting the music must be for him," referring to Hanks' character. She was consoling me at the same time.

After watching the film, four of us were interviewed for our reactions. Our comments accompanied the film's review the next day. Sid summarized the reality of the experience: "In the last six weeks, I have said goodbye to a person in a hospital bed knowing I was not going to see him again. And trying to find the words to say goodbye to someone is everything I saw on that screen." Mark Siwiec, of the Gay and Lesbian

"'YOU'RE THE AIDS DOCTOR. YOU ARE RESPONSIBLE NOT ONLY FOR WHAT YOU SAY BUT FOR WHAT PEOPLE HEAR.'"

Political Caucus, captured the essence of the fight and said, "So much of what we're all fighting for was in this one film." Cora Mancuso, whose son Fred died the year before, said that not all people with AIDS were Philadelphia lawyers. She reminded us not to forget the little guy.

My comments were on-script. The voice of my mentor, Bob Loeb, echoed in my brain: "You're the AIDS doctor. You are responsible for not only what you say but for what people hear." So, telling the reporter how painful this film was for me personally would be off the mark. I went with a more global message, saying that this film might help "re-shape" some attitudes about AIDS and what a slow process that was.

Jack Garner, the local newspaper's film critic, agreed. In his review, he chastised the Hollywood establishment for taking so long to bring a story about AIDS to the screen.

There was one more event planned by Sid that continued the tradition of eating and playing together to survive. This time we were saying *bon voyage* to our friend and co-founder of CHN, Dr. Steve Scheibel, who was moving to San Francisco to launch the next phase of his career.

Sid often included clinic people on the invitation list for the elegant yet comfortable buffet suppers at the Metzger home. This time, she outdid herself and planned a "Biker Chic" party. The inspiration—Scheibel's biker style.

Steve, known for his brain and equally impressive well-toned body, usually wore biker garb to the office. Black T, jeans, and motorcycle boots completed the outfit. And, his wallet on a chain. The party invitation encouraged people to wear biker black in honor of Steve. And they did.

In our usual style, we worked hard and played hard—not only for ourselves but for the benefit of our patients.

Though Sid is gone, her memory lingers. Rest well, Sid, for a job well done.

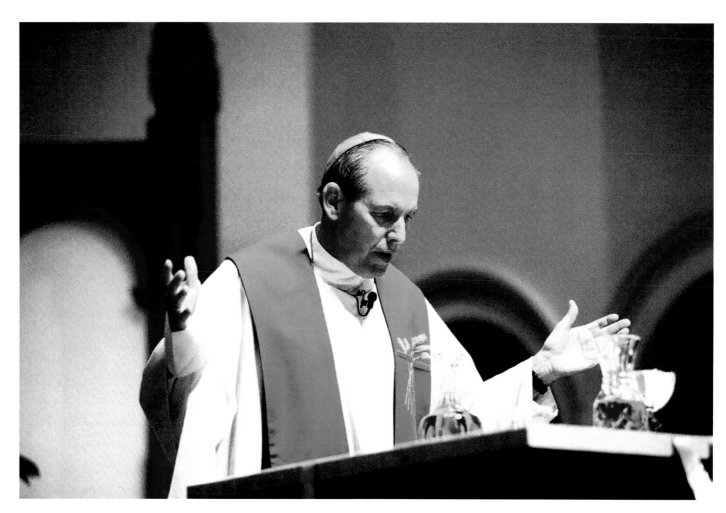

▸ Bishop Matthew H. Clark celebrates mass at Rochester's St. Mary's Church, September 19, 1998 at the annual conference of the National Association of Catholic Lesbian and Gay Ministries. His ministry was transformational and helped restore the faith of many of us.

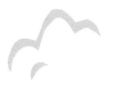

13 | DAYDREAMS: FAITH RESTORED

There hasn't been a day since 1981 when I haven't spent a good
part of it thinking about some aspect or other of HIV.

I daydream a lot. Occasionally, I pass my exit on the highway while driving as a result. Usually one, sometimes two exits, so I never go too far out of my way. Once in a while, I am late for meetings. To avoid missed flights, I leave way too early for the airport. While I have missed plenty of exits, I have missed only one flight in my life.

I daydreamed in church as a child. I suppose I should have been defining my faith, but I was distracted. Instead, I used the time to formulate ideas and reflect on the goings-on in my 7-year-old life.

One major distraction was a girl in my class, Carla, who disappeared from school in first grade when she contracted polio. She came back to church a year later wearing a heavy leg brace. I could hear her clanking brace before I saw her, and then I watched her walk behind her family as they made their way to the front of the church. I imagine my mother was equally distracted. Her sister was a polio survivor, so the impact of polio was also a family matter.

My adult daydreams are generally productive. They usually have something to do with HIV care: a particular patient, something a patient told me, the healthcare system, something I've read about HIV, something I'm working on currently, how to string the words together in a presentation I'm preparing.

I rehearse a talk I'm giving or what I will say in a media interview. I like to look like I am doing these things off the cuff, so I try to memorize what I'm going to say. It works pretty well most of the time, unless, of course, I miss my exit on the highway.

I remember driving to work one time when early intervention solidified in my mind. Steve Scheibel and I had been talking about it for years, so the idea was always on my mind. During that drive in 1986, while we were still testing AZT in a clinical trial, it all came together. I realized that we should use AZT and treat people earlier, rather than waiting until T-cells fell below 200, the patient's immune system was exhausted, and there was less chance of recovery. That was a novel idea, or so I thought. Today, I wonder if we were on the leading edge or if the idea was just hiding in plain sight.

I had been serving on the AIDS Institute's Standards of Care Committee since it was formed in 1984 and continue to do so today. I went to a committee meeting after AZT was approved and offered my view on early treatment. My colleagues weren't ready for that, and, for the life of me, I couldn't understand it.

In retrospect, I get it now. Most of the group was from New York City, and the situation was far more desperate in the city. We were dealing with small numbers in Rochester—in the hundreds. In New York City, the number of patients was in the thousands. So, our Rochester version of early intervention was logistically impossible in New York City at the time.

I didn't re-evaluate myself from a faith perspective until 1988. I was moved by Rochester Catholic Bishop Matthew Clark's "Pastoral Letter" to the community. His 30-page letter urged compassion and called faithful people to action to address the growing number of people in the community with AIDS. Nine years later, he held a mass for gay, lesbian, bisexual, and transgender people that was standing-room-only. This was followed a year later with a mass for people with AIDS, their families, and their caregivers.

I remember the evening mass for people with AIDS. In contrast to my childhood distraction at mass, they had my rapt attention. I can still see the Bishop entering the nave, the central aisle, of the church. The pageantry and symbolism of what was happening moved me to tears. I finally understood what might make people fall to their knees during these experiences.

Though I remained standing, it was the personal awakening I had been waiting for and needed so badly. We all needed it, and, personally, I felt some relief from the huge load that had been on my shoulders. Finally, my own faith had been moved to a higher level.

Carol Williams remembered that mass. She said, "there was healing in the air." She also described the power of prayer that got her through those days. She tells the story of her daughter, Amy, who died at the age of 10 months after cardiac surgery. After a lot of reflection, Carol believes that she did AIDS work as part of her recovery from Amy's death many years earlier; Amy was her messenger. She wanted Amy's short life to have meaning and translated her grief into service to others. She also observed that my

"MY MESSENGERS HAVE BEEN HIDING IN PLAIN SIGHT ALL THESE YEARS ... "

classmate Carla, like her Amy, was my messenger.

Carol saw the obvious here. I failed to recognize it until Carol said that Carla has God's messenger written all over her. I would add another messenger to my list—my mother's sister, my Aunt Ellen, who survived polio as a child. While the residual effects from her polio (she refused to use the term disability) were not as profound as Carla's, she still had guts and determination. She was an important and pivotal part of my life.

My messengers have been hiding in plain sight all these years; I just failed to recognize them until now. Carol said it recently when she described her definition of faith—you can't see it, but you believe it.

Steve Scheibel's faith was formed as a child, not with traditional religion but, instead, by developing what he describes as a broad, deep worldview. I've always known Steve to be a deep thinker. Recently, he explained the depth of his thinking and the link to his spiritual side. His worldview encompasses a connection between spiritual, mental, and physical health.

While I have always known him to be a risk taker, he is a calculated risk taker. Obviously, this worldview translates into his care of patients. Recently, he explained to me how he filters out the risk or bad energy to make rational, science-based decisions that are not only ahead of the curve but safe for patients. In other words, his spiritual and scientific sides are linked, and his spirituality informs the science. He doesn't just pull ideas out of his head. There's more to it.

His instincts are grounded in science and have been refined over time. It was only natural that he would arrive at early intervention for HIV care before anyone else. While we were doing early intervention in the 1980s, it would be another 30 years before the global scientific community's standard of care would be to treat everyone with HIV as soon as possible. While the early intervention battle has finally been put to rest, Steve still reads 20 scientific articles a day to keep up.

We weren't alone with this idea. There were many other iconoclasts struggling with the same idea globally. While we were refining the idea of early intervention, we were trying to balance the risk with science and, as I have come to appreciate, with spirituality. In the end, I think everyone knew that this was the right way to do HIV care. We just came to the realization at different times in different ways.

The common denominator was that all of us were torn. We struggled with the need for more drugs to treat HIV, pushing the envelope using the available drugs and trying to keep patients from accessing dangerous treatments that were available through the underground.

Thankfully, our patients and their families, in an expression of their faith in us, followed our advice.

WILLIAM M. VALENTI, M.D.

*Supporting the development of Community
Health Network is among my favorite memories
and a highlight of my career.*

—Arthur Collier, Chief Operating Officer, Rochester
Primary Care Network, now Regional Primary Care
Network, Rochester, New York

14 | RYAN WHITE: HIS LEGACY OF HEALTHCARE AND ADVOCACY

The contagion wars reached fever pitch in 1985 when Ryan White, an Indiana teenager with AIDS, was denied admission to school. The legal battles that followed were divisive and embarrassing for me to watch.

We were finally settled into our new clinic space and were consumed with patient care. Then the realization hit. We were doctors, and we were also running a business. Words like cash flow, payroll, accounting and bookkeeping, insurance, compliance, and grant reporting were forced into our vocabulary. Where was the money?

We needed an executive director to manage our finances, and eventually we hired a man who had retired from a local health organization. The financial picture proved too distressing for him. One Saturday morning, after a month on the job, he called me at home and submitted his resignation, effective immediately. I was back in the driver's seat. After I called Peggy Clark, our board chair, and Steve Scheibel, I did something I rarely do when I'm stressed. I climbed into bed, pulled the covers over my head, and took a nap in the middle of the day.

Cash flow was very slow, as Dr. Nick Rango had predicted. We were broke. Nancy Adams, executive director of the Monroe County Medical Society, persuaded a retiring physician to donate an exam table, supplies, and a copier. Prone to breakdowns, the copier included an extended warranty. One day, the copier repairman came and said the service call was included in the warranty, but he needed $15 for parts. I had $2 in my wallet. Remember, we were taking patients regardless of ability to pay. When we opened, we framed our first co-pays from patients: a $5 and a $10 bill. I took the money out of the frame, copied the bills on the newly repaired copier, and put the copy of the money back in the frame. I gave the real $15 to the repairman.

Austerity budget took on a new meaning. Board members shared the cost of food for our evening meetings. For every meeting for the first several years, my mother sent a tray of her butter cookies for dessert. Dr. Charlie Solky, psychiatrist and board member, loved my mother's baked goods, so Mom made a point of sending a package of extra cookies for him to take home.

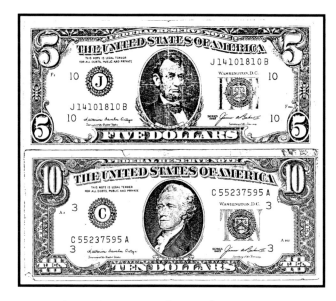

▶ Framed copy of co-payments from our first two patients. The real bills were used to pay for copier repairs.

He sent her a note from time to time, and she would gush over the attention.

It was fortuitous that early in our planning phase, I had described the idea of an AIDS clinic to John Urban, the head of the Preferred Care HMO, now MVP Health Care. Urban introduced me to Art Collier, president of the Rochester Primary Care Network, a federally-funded consortium of community health centers. Collier and I connected instantly. An iconoclast at heart, he loved the CHN idea. I paid him $1 for CHN to join RPCN as a member agency. That was a dollar well spent, because the return on this meager investment made it possible for us to sustain the work at CHN in the start-up years. Perhaps the most significant act that gave us a critical boost that we needed to stay afloat was working with Art to write our first federal Ryan White Care Act grant. It was funded in 1990, the first year of the Ryan White program's existence.

Ryan White, the Indiana teenager, was one of the early hemophilia patients with AIDS. He made an indelible mark on the movement as he and his mother courageously fought to allow him to stay in school. Fear of contagion was a huge flashpoint in those days. The stigma extended beyond school. Customers on White's paper route canceled their subscriptions as threats of violence and lawsuits continued. Ryan White became the icon of a movement to educate people about the human rights issues for people with AIDS. Ryan died in 1990 at the age of 18. His legacy lives on in the federal Ryan White Care Act that continues to fund HIV care throughout the U.S.

Several weeks or months after we submitted the grant, Art called with "urgent news" while I was seeing patients. "Write down $165,500," he exclaimed. As I was writing, he said, "That's your Ryan White grant. Congratulations. Now get back to work." First, there were hugs with the team, and then there was the realization of what this meant for patients. No more worrying about how to pay for their care. We were ahead of the epidemic for five minutes.

Collier and Neal Garver, then our director of operations, launched the Ryan White grant. During Garver's time with us, we came close to breaking even financially.

When Dan Holland, another risk-taker, took over as executive director, he brought in administrative people to take care of our growing business. Holland was calm, collected, and a gentleman. Though we still ran a deficit, he deserves the credit for putting systems in place that we lacked. Two notable hires were Barb DiMarco, executive assistant, and Arlene VanHalle, who did purchasing, facilities management, and "everything else."

Barb, after 26 years on staff, has the title of "Employee 002." We laugh at the thought of how far we've come. Other long-timers include Doug Lindke and Mark Malahosky, pharmacists and also Melinda Sents and Rich Fowler. Collectively, we have more than 150 years of service.

On the other side of town, Paula Silvestrone became the new executive director of AIDS Rochester (ARI) in 1990. While we took care of patients, Paula, ably assisted by Michael Beatty and Annie Long, was going head-to-head with the district attorney over ARI's plan for a clean-needle exchange. Some people in the community connected needle exchange with encouraging drug use. Today, needle exchange has helped control the epidemic in injection drug users. Paula would also open two ARI service offices, one in Bath, New York, and one in Geneva, New York, that extended ARI's reach to rural areas. Later, Paula and Jay Rudman, then CEO of AIDS Care (formerly CHN), saw the wisdom of a merger of the two organizations— the foundation for today's Trillium Health.

By 1990, at the CHN clinic on South Avenue, our clinical pharmacy initiative had started with the assistance of Dr. Rodney Voisine. Dr. Rodney was a friend, supporter, patient advocate, and a very smart guy. A natural networker, we met several years earlier when he appeared unannounced in clinic during his residency interviews to introduce himself.

His degrees in medicine and pharmacy helped us sort out the never-ending list of natural supplements and purported "antivirals" that our patients presented us with. He continued to volunteer on his post call days to give us some relief. In retrospect, we had developed one of the first clinical pharmacy programs anywhere.

Years later, he reminded me of our frequent discussions that, eventually, HIV would be treated as a chronic disease. Along with us, the global mix of advocates, volunteers, and dedicated people on the front lines would see to it. Still, amidst the chaos, I never imagined that we would be talking today about ending the HIV epidemic.

Once the clinic was buzzing, I could get out of town occasionally. Art Collier had friends in high places in the Ryan White program and dispatched me to Washington, D.C. to do the keynote address at the first Ryan White National Conference in 1991. When he gave me the "good news," I asked, "What should I tell them? That the two drugs we have both stink? What else?" He said, "Tell them about early intervention. They need to know how to run an AIDS program." I wasn't sure the audience would understand our brand of early intervention, but I agreed to do the talk.

I spoke to about 500 people on "The Future of AIDS Care." I was introduced by Dr. Merle Cunningham, who would become a lifelong friend, colleague, and mentor. I told the audience that we needed more money to fund treatment and research—that when we had more drugs, early intervention would get legs.

I droned on and on. I showed a busy, unreadable slide of how to treat the AIDS opportunistic infections. As I looked out at the audience, many had a glazed look on their faces. I wasn't connecting with them. Collier was right. They were newbies and had just begun the fight. As a Niagara Falls of perspiration soaked my back and armpits, I saw that people were leaving. I looked at Cunningham, who cocked his head and raised his eyebrows as if to say, "You're taking on water. Do something to save this."

I decided to go off-script and into advocacy mode. I went on, "We need to do something about AIDS stigma and fight the fear of contagion," I

nearly shouted. "Ryan White couldn't go to school! When Ronald Reagan was president, he never even mentioned the word AIDS! What kind of crap is that?" I thought about saying "bullshit" but couldn't bring myself to do it. The audience responded. Some stood up, applauded, hooted, and stamped their feet. I went on to say, "The only person in the Reagan administration who made sense was Surgeon General Koop who defied conservatives and sent a pamphlet on *Understanding AIDS* to every house in the United States in 1986."

Koop, a conservative evangelical, had been directed by administration advisors to condemn homosexuality in his pamphlet. Instead, he took his duty as the nation's doctor seriously. This thoughtful educational piece said, "We are fighting a disease, not people," a classic message for a desperate era.

I thanked the audience for their enthusiastic response and left to call the office to check in with Steve. There were no cell phones in those days, so I called from a phone booth in the hotel lobby. Steve told me that one of our patients had been admitted to Highland the day before and had toxoplasmosis of the brain, another disabling opportunistic infection.

I felt like someone had hit me over the head with a very big hammer. I had just shown the slide that addressed this, unreadable as it was. I thought I was a hopeless failure. Why didn't we see this coming? We went on to treat his infection, but he had a difficult time with frequent hospitalizations until he died two years later. Fortunately, his family was there for him and fought with him until the end.

We would learn a year later in 1992, that people with CD4 (T-cells) less than 200 were at risk for what we were calling "opportunistic infections." At that point, we were still shooting in the dark with managing patients and trying to prevent these infections. After that breakthrough, we covered people with low CD4 cells with every preventive drug available. Most treatment guidelines hadn't addressed this yet, so we created our own until the guidelines caught up.

The era highlights the old adage: "You don't know what you don't know." Our approach at the time now validates our style of making up the rules as we went along. What we were doing was creating the evidence, although we didn't know

that at the time either. If we had failed to act, our slow progress would have been even slower.

As I was heading out the door of the hotel to catch my plane, I ran into Michael Callen, the AIDS activist from New York, who said, "Nice job, doc. You got their attention with that Reagan comment!"

During our quick conversation in Washington, he said something that has stayed with me all these years. "Doc, this is my life's work. It's all I think about," he said. That resonated with me. I felt the same way. That's all I thought about and still do.

As I tried to doze on the flight home, I thought about our local activist, Tony Green, who was constantly telling the political establishment, "We need more drugs—NOW!" Maybe I should join the advocates in protest, I thought. I imagined myself helping tear down the AZT manufacturer's display booth at the next international conference. The pace is too slow. We need to do more—and do it better! And faster!

With or without me, these protests certainly got people's attention at major AIDS conferences. In fact, it was the AIDS activist movement that moved the FDA to make experimental drugs available before their final approval under what we were now calling "Early Access."

When I woke up in Rochester, I deplaned and headed to Highland to see my patient.

Fast forward to the modern era: Our Trillium intake coordinator came into my office recently. She wanted some advice about our consent form to treat a 17-year-old young man whose mother called, wanting us to treat her son with the once-a-day HIV prevention pill (PrEP). I asked her, "What would you rather do—see this high-risk kid become HIV-positive while we figure out if this is the correct consent form? Or would you rather just do it and have his mom sign this form." She responded instantly, "Do it," and left the room. All perfectly legal, only faster. I wanted to hug her.

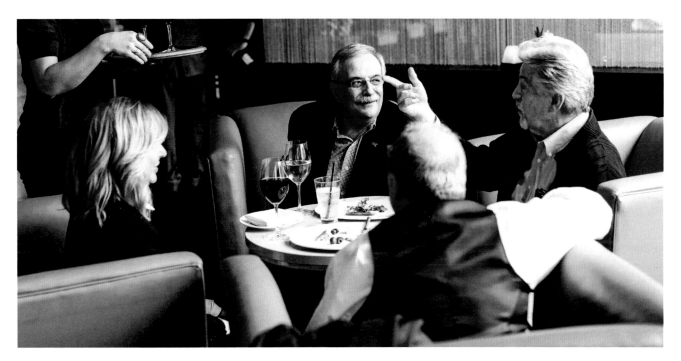

▸ Dr. Merle Cunningham makes a point 26 years later as we listen with rapt attention. Clockwise from far left: Andrea DeMeo, president, Trillium Health; Bill Valenti; Merle Cunningham; and another of Merle's long-time colleagues, Peter Robinson, chief operating officer, University of Rochester Medical Center. 2016. Merle died unexpectedly in 2016 leaving a legacy to LGBTQ health and the community health center movement.

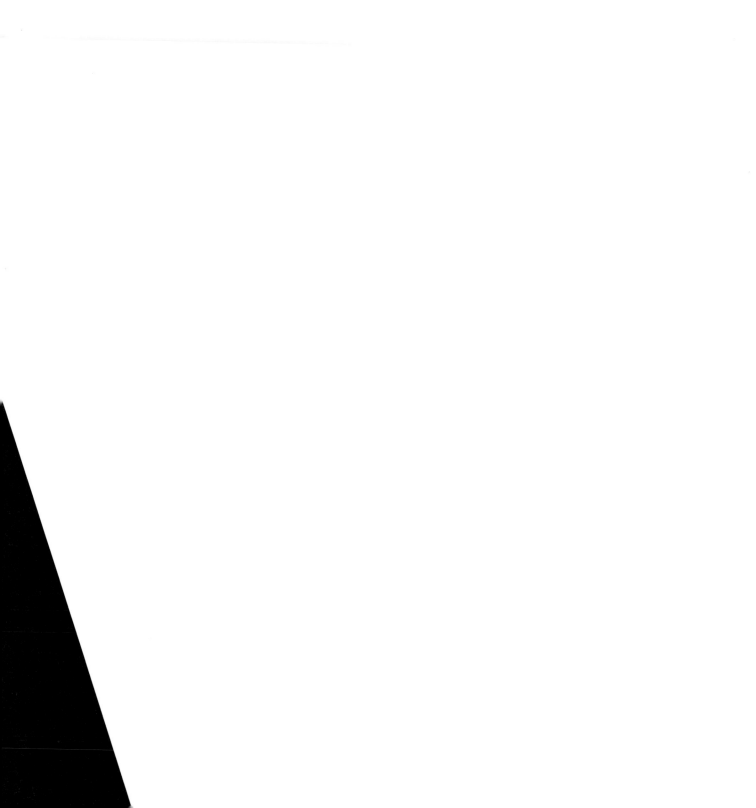

15 | OUT OF THE DARK

I knew enough not to blame myself for his blindness. Still, I second-guessed my decisions, thinking that if only we had done something different, this might not have happened. At the same time, I didn't know what the "something different" should have been.

Blindness resulting from cytomegalovirus (CMV) infection was devastating and overwhelming. In addition to Kaposi's sarcoma, it was another cruel opportunistic complication of AIDS.

As I reflect, I've asked myself what would you rather have—Kaposi's that scarred your body with terrible purple spots? Or, would you rather be blind from CMV? There were no good choices here. The whole scene became a race to try and stay ahead of these terrible infections. Most of the time, especially in this early era, we struggled to keep up.

One day in 1991, an early patient, a talented artist, came in for his appointment. I can still see us sitting across from each other and talking in an exam room. I have never forgotten his words. All of a sudden, he said, "I can't see. It's like a window shade came over my eyes. Everything's dark."

I felt helpless. I jumped up and guided him to the exam table. I looked in his eyes with the ophthalmoscope immediately and saw what I

"WE NOW HAD A PATIENT WHO DROVE HIMSELF TO THE OFFICE AND, OVER THE COURSE OF A FEW HOURS, WENT BLIND."

thought were the characteristic "cotton wool" spots of CMV. We dispatched him to the emergency department and admitted him, but it was too late. The ophthalmologist confirmed the spots of CMV retinitis. He was treated but never recovered his vision.

The next day, Steve Scheibel and I reviewed the situation with chief nurse Carol Williams and Sid Metzger, social worker. Second-guessing myself didn't help. We now had a patient who drove himself to the office and, over the course of a few hours, went blind. And now he was a

blind artist. I was numbed by the relentlessness of the whole experience.

Later, I thought, "What next? Can't we catch a break here for a minute?" The answer was always the same. Scheibel's battle cry, "We push ahead. The work is too important not to."

So, now we had two blind patients who used canes to get around—two blind and very courageous patients, I might add. As a result of the experiences with these two patients, we launched the "Eye Watch" program in which all patients had quarterly eye exams with retina photographs. Early intervention, once again, would carry the day.

For the record, a volunteer group of dedicated eye doctors made this program happen. A pet project of Art Collier, the Eye Watch program was funded initially by the Rochester Primary Care Network. The concept was simple, yet revolutionary for the time. The idea was to identify CMV retinitis as early as possible by detecting its telltale spots on an eye exam and starting treatment early to prevent blindness. Once this well-oiled program was launched, we had no more blind patients.

Southside Apothecary was our pharmacy partner and maintained a pick-up station at CHN. Pharmacists Mark Malahosky and Doug Lindke were part of this early pharmacy revolution, working at their headquarters in the high-tech pharmacy that our pharmacy partner set up in response to the demand. Mark said recently, "I never really got over to the Community Health Network office very much in those days. It seemed like we were always mixing the drugs for CMV treatment—we never left the prep room. It was insane."

Lisa Brozek, our infusion nurse, did the intravenous treatments, both in the CHN office and in patients' homes. The demand was high, and she was another one-person force of nature. Also a multitasker, she was energetic and passionate about the work. She would fly into the office, greet everyone with a smile, get a patient started on treatment, write chart notes, talk on the phone, and head out to do a home visit.

She visited us at Trillium Health recently and recalled, "It was like a war zone during that era. One day ran into the next!" In another discussion, she talked about her patients. Once again, as she spoke, I could see their faces. Steve Scheibel echoed my sentiments another time when he said he could still identify his early patients by name and see their faces.

Thankfully, CMV retinitis disappeared in the early 1990s with the introduction of a triple-drug combination therapy for HIV. Drs. Thomas Ophardt and Kevin Wynne have the distinction of having put this baby to bed by identifying the last cases of CMV retinitis anywhere. Gone. Done. Goodbye.

Despite the intensity, fast pace, and relentlessness of the experience, we all managed to pull together. The end game? These innovators saved the vision of thousands of people.

In my book, they were nothing short of heroic.

16 | CHRISTINE'S BROTHERS

Many patients came home to be with family when they
were too sick to manage on their own. Fortunately, Jim and
Larry had their sister Christine who rose to the challenge.

I remember both Jim and Larry Fritsch very well. Both had moved back home from New York City in the late 1980s: Larry first, then Jim six months later. Jim was the jovial brother with the infectious laugh. In New York, he wanted to be a Broadway star. An aspiring actor, he did have a bit part in the movie *Yanks* with Vanessa Redgrave. When he came back home, he refocused his acting career, taking on many roles in plays about HIV/AIDS. Though infected with HIV, he was determined to live out his life's dream on the local Rochester scene. He became a star of the Shipping Dock Theatre.

Larry was quieter and more serious than his brother, Jim. With his dark, serious good looks, he headed to New York City with a goal of becoming a model. But that remained an unfulfilled dream. He lived in Greenwich Village, was a student at NYU, and became a

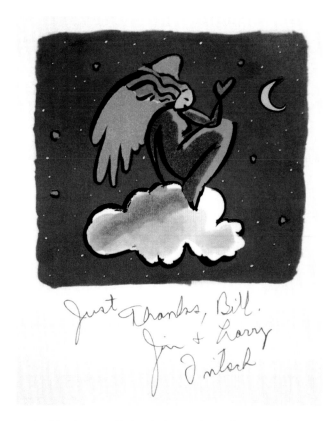

▶ Jim Fritsch wrote this inscription on the inside cover of the book.

graphic designer. He worked for *Arts and Antiques* magazine.

Steve and Carol took care of Larry. I was Jim's doctor. One day, Jim presented a gift to me in an exam room during one of his office visits. Beautifully wrapped, I can still see his smile as

I pulled out *The Angel Book* by Karen Goldman. "Maybe this will help you with your job," he said. "I could never do what you do."

Jim took care of Larry through his dying days, knowing full well what his fate would be. And then, six months later, he, too, would die. AIDS robbed the Fritsch family of not only Jim and Larry but their cousin as well.

Their sister Christine, along with her partner, the late Nina Miller, grateful for the care we provided for her brothers at CHN, became a voice for supporting the fight against AIDS and has been a regular donor since Jim and Larry died.

Christine wrote the letter below 20 years later, in 2014. She recalled her experiences and expressed the feelings of many families affected by AIDS during that era.

Why Do I Give?

When I bought my house in the South Wedge down the street from CHN on South Ave. in 1989, little did I know what an important role CHN would play in my family's life.

My youngest brother, Larry, returned to Rochester from New York City when he was diagnosed with HIV. His illness progressed to

AIDS, and he passed away in December 1993. Another brother, Jim, came home from NYC several months later. Also diagnosed with AIDS, he passed away in June 1994. Both brothers made their base at my home and received their medical care at CHN.

Dr. Bill Valenti and Sid Metzger were invaluable medical, informational, and emotional supports for both my brothers and our family throughout several years of heart-breaking physical illness, treatments, and hospitalizations. They will always have my unending love and gratitude for their part in my brothers' lives.

Following my brothers' deaths, as part of my own grief and eventual healing, I began giving personal financial backing and encouraged others to contribute to CHN. I started a team of teachers, staff, and friends at #4 School in the city, where I was a Special Education teacher, to participate in the annual AIDS Walks. We raised several thousand dollars each year for 10 years.

For the past 20 years I followed the transitions from CHN to AIDS Care to Trillium Health. I continue to follow research breakthroughs with interest, encourage financial *support, and maintain thankfulness and respect for organizations like Trillium Health.*

Christine's letter captures the essence of the impact of AIDS on families. In this case, she describes a "homecoming" experience. Typical of the era, many young men came home from larger cities, especially New York City, when they were sick and needed medical care.

She describes the connection to our staff, a lifeline for families during that difficult era. Imagine the lives interrupted and the pain of having three people in your family dying at the height of their careers. Fortunately, Larry and Jim had a loving sister who stepped up to the plate.

WILLIAM M. VALENTI, M.D.

Losing a patient was painful enough to face as a caregiver. After all these years, I still find it difficult to reconcile how this must have felt for families.

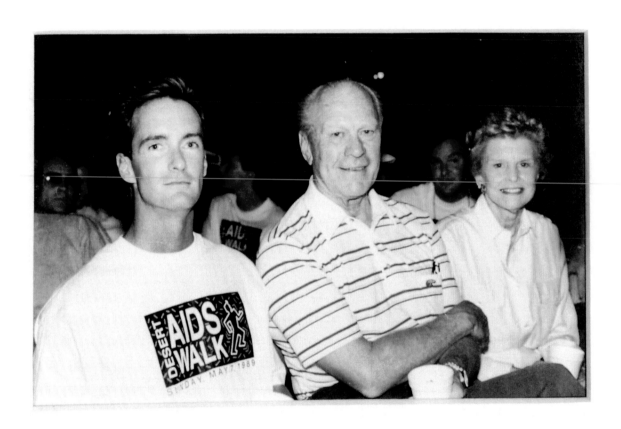

▸ Bud Shaw with President Gerald Ford and First Lady Betty Ford, Palm Springs, 1985.

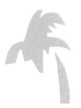

17 | THE MAN FROM PALM SPRINGS: DONALD "BUD" SHAW

Bud told me that he liked networking and using
his quiet influence to raise money for the cause.

Donald "Bud" Shaw, Jr., like many of my patients, was a Rochester native. He had a confident, low-key personality. With patrician looks just out of central casting, he was articulate, passionate, and generous. He was also very smart, and I liked the way he looked at things strategically.

Bud had been a major force raising money for the Desert AIDS Project in Palm Springs. His brother, Bernard "Barney" Shaw, liked to tell the story of how the Desert AIDS Project had a low budget with a $20,000 deficit when Bud arrived. By the time he left, the organization had a $1.8 million endowment and 14 employees.

When he came home from Palm Springs, we were located in our newly opened clinic on South Avenue. In fact, he worked for us as a volunteer in our understaffed development program for a while. He and our social worker, Sid Metzger, developed a fast friendship.

The two had endless conversations about books, theater, medical care, and fundraising.

My conversations with Bud centered around conquering AIDS. In one of our conversations, he said that he had accepted a world *with* AIDS, but his goal was to see a world without it. And, regarding his fundraising prowess, he said he wanted to do his part. He liked connecting the dots.

We have photos of Bud with President Gerald Ford and former First Lady Betty Ford with a note from Betty wishing him well in his efforts, and photos of him with the actor Kirk Douglas and his wife Anne. In other words, Bud was a powerhouse when it came to promoting AIDS organizations and raising money.

In early 1992, he became the honorary chair of one of our early fundraising events. "An Event in Three Acts" was on a U.S. tour sponsored by the Design Industry Foundation for AIDS (DIFFA). This show has been called the most successful AIDS fundraiser ever, raising millions. Still, it was a bit risky, considering the short lead-time. He worked tirelessly to help put it together with Ken Maldonado, our development director at the time.

Sadly, Bud died in March 1992 and never saw the success of his last in a long series of good works. We dedicated the event to him. I remember the excitement and energy of opening night, May 23, 1992, at the Auditorium Theater

"THAT NIGHT, CHRISTINE KLOS PROVIDED THE ANCHOR I NEEDED TO GET BEYOND THE ANXIETY OF PULLING THIS OFF."

in Rochester. I scanned the long line of guests waiting to enter the auditorium as anxious as an expectant father. I locked eyes with Dave and Christine Klos and was comforted by Christine's smile and her offer of "Congratulations!" We smooched, and I hugged our then-pharmacy partner Dave Klos. I had met Christine years earlier at Strong Memorial, so we had a history together. That night, Christine provided the anchor I needed to get beyond the anxiety of pulling this off. We did it, and we basked in the glow of our success.

Parts two and three of this extravaganza included The AIDS Walk and a showing of the AIDS Memorial Quilt in May and June, respectively. Event four, a bonus, was the Helping People with AIDS fundraiser in September 1992.

An Event in Three Acts was a tremendous financial success, once again demonstrating the synergy between the community and the AIDS effort. Thankfully, An Event in Three Acts helped to pave the way for future fundraising events for our AIDS efforts in Rochester.

During his two years in Rochester, Bud and his supportive family were passionate about the work we were doing. They became a part of our family of patients, advocates, providers, staff, and community partners.

When Bud died, in addition to his bequest to CHN, he distributed the remainder of his estate to his nine nieces and nephews. He stipulated that by the time they were 30 years old, they needed to donate their inheritance to the charity of their choice. To honor their uncle, they donated those bequests to CHN to create two conference rooms and a comfortable waiting area that we use for mental health patients. The area has been named after the Shaw Family in perpetuity.

At the dedication, his family wrote a joint remembrance of Bud. Some of their thoughts were that "deep within Buddy came a love of ceremony, a flair for the extravagant, and a flawless attention to detail." Hidden beneath all of that was a soul that loved to laugh and help others. More than anything, Bud liked to give the party, be at the center of the party, and be remembered longest after the party. Beyond his attention to detail, he was a faithful and loyal friend.

In another remembrance of Bud, his brother Barney talked about Bud's last days and focused on a call to action. At the dedication of the Shaw Family space in Bud's memory, he said that we all "can make a big difference to the Buds of the future. Fundraising activities like An Event in Three Acts help provide the best medical care available and the best social support and education."

At our Trillium Health office, we have appropriated one of the donated rooms for our information technology and business intelligence staff. Bud would be pleased to know that we are using the Shaw Family space strategically.

He and his family continue to help us pay attention to detail, connect the dots, and end the epidemic.

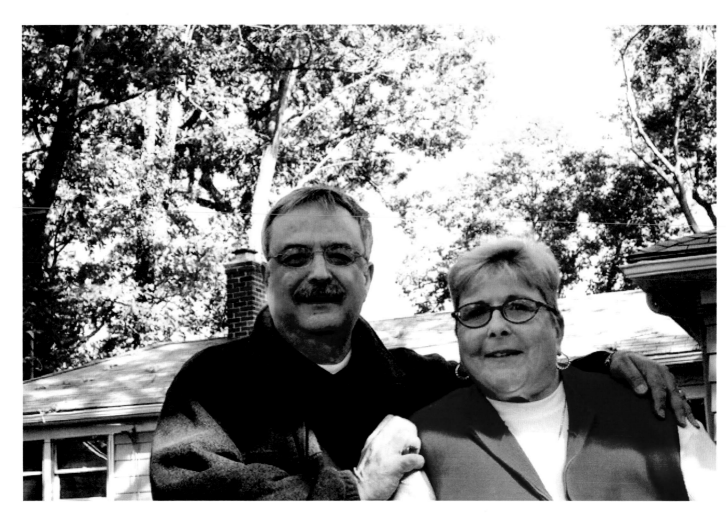

▸ Bill Valenti and Toni Obermeyer, 2006.

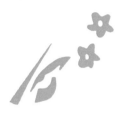

18 | IF YOU MAKE THE RULES, YOU CAN BREAK THE RULES: TONI OBERMEYER

Fact and fantasy often became blurred when the three of us were together, giving rise to the concept of one-stop shopping for the comprehensive treatment of HIV/AIDS.

— Dr. Steven Scheibel

Toni Obermeyer: June 14, 1949–January 27, 2007

We were all reeling from the sudden death of our friend and colleague, Toni. It was so unexpected. Tone's children, Felice and York, asked me to speak at her memorial service.

It was held at Blessed Sacrament Church in Rochester and was packed with the people she had touched. Before I spoke, soprano Jackie Jester Castiglia, Tone's friend and our former CHN office assistant, sang Schubert's "Ave Maria." For the second time in a decade, I was reduced to tears in church.

I told the audience that Jackie was a tough act to follow. Then, I read prepared remarks, because I knew I could not do this one without a script.

It is very difficult, if not impossible, to capture the essence of Toni Obermeyer in a few words. Also known as Toni O, The Tone, Tone, and my personal favorite, Tone-a-Rama, the bigger-than-life Tone. A colorful character, if ever there was one. The following is a letter I read at the service called "Oh Toni, Toni O":

Dear Tone,

We'll miss you. You certainly left in a hurry. That's not like you to arrive or leave unannounced like that. Somehow we thought you were indestructible and would be here much longer. The good news, of course, is that where you are there are no more pills to take. You can also watch your favorite movie for all eternity: George Cukor's 1939 classic *The Women*.

Our Meeting

We first met when I lost my wallet and your son, York, found it lying in the street in October 1985.

York tracked me down, and when I went to pick up my wallet at your house, the money and credit cards were still inside. At that meeting,

York said, in what was surely an understatement, "You should meet my mother." At the time, you were working as the Home Care Coordinator for HIV patients at a local agency. When we met a few days later, I had no idea of the adventures that lay ahead. Thank you, York, for your integrity and for that introduction.

Making Up the Rules as You Go Along

One of the reasons we got along so well was that we were both impatient for action, and we often did an end run around any obstacles to get the job done.

In the early days of the AIDS epidemic, we were all flying by the seat of our pants doing things that had never been done before. You were front and center with that. During your two years at AIDS Rochester, you put HIV street outreach on the map.

I can see your picture on the front page of the B section of the evening paper around 1989. You were standing in the doorway of a crack house, getting ready to charge upstairs and work with people to get them straight through drug treatment and HIV testing. You talked about harm reduction and "meeting people where they are" long before it became established as a standard of care.

After Community Health Network opened in 1989, you brought people to the office for testing or to be enrolled in care—street outreach that linked people to care. "You need to know street lingo," you once told us. So, you gave us a glossary of street terms "so that you know what people are talking about."

Steve Scheibel recalls: "I learned so much from Toni. She had so many different life experiences from which to draw. She worked hard to make me, the gay white boy from the Midwest, understand. Bleach kits, clean works, shooting galleries, ghettos, the projects, and sex work were some of her 'preachin'' topics. We walked the streets and did outreach to help stem HIV infections in injection drug users. Toni watched over me carefully, knowing that, in my ignorance, I would always prove to be too white."

The New York Experience

Later, after your elopement with the man from Morocco, you moved to Belle Harbor, New York, that sandbar on the Atlantic, and commuted to work in the substance abuse program at Albert Einstein Medical College in the Bronx. There, your street outreach was like a fast-moving train. Your supervisor recalled to me that, "Toni and the Bronx were made for each other."

Later, you had your own mobile clinic, working for The Foundation for Research on Sexually Transmitted Diseases. The van did outreach to sex workers in Lower New York, and you supervised the residential program.

When you moved to a bigger stage at the AIDS Institute in the state health department, you shook things up there for another year. Your supervisor there noted, "I've never met anyone quite like Toni!"

Outside of work, we covered a lot of territory in New York. Remember the night we saw Eartha Kitt's show at the Café Carlyle? Lucky Chang's restaurant on the Lower East Side was your find. All of the servers were Asian men in drag, and the house dessert was a chocolate high-heeled shoe filled with chocolate mousse. We ate the whole shoe.

I enjoyed our bohemian days drinking cheap wine from plastic cups on the balcony at the Chelsea Hotel on West 23rd Street. Okay, it wasn't exactly a balcony. It was the fire escape.

I was relieved when we graduated to the Gramercy Park Hotel; it was a bit more civilized in its own shabby, 2½-star way. At least we could get breakfast in the hotel. Another reason why we got along so well was that you could be enthusiastic about scrambled eggs at 7 in the morning or 7 at night. And I never went into your house when there wasn't a pot of coffee brewing. Those small things make a big difference.

Expecting the Unexpected

I remember the party you hosted at my house. You asked if you could invite a few people over to listen to music. I was out of town and missed the event. The house was spotless when I returned, and I never would have guessed that your small party consisted of 100 guests and a reggae band. You were very reassuring when you told me that "at least no one was arrested. Besides, Ann Zettelmaier was there to keep an eye on things!"

In any event, things like that could never damage a good friendship, including one of your visits when you brought some laundry to do. What's a blown-out washing machine motor between friends anyway? Our friendship outlasted all of that, including a few of my own personal relationships that began and ended during our friendship.

Steve Scheibel summed up your friendship this way: "A friend is the sum of all the experiences, thoughts, and feelings you ever have. It is not bound by the past, present, or future. I remember Tone's cottage on Gregory Street, hanging out with her kids Felice and York and Ethel, the basset hound, in the chill of a Rochester winter that just wouldn't go away. I see us walking across an empty lot dotted with soot-tinged snow and limp grass, engrossed in conversation about some aspect of AIDS or other, and shedding tears for those we had lost to the epidemic. With Toni, the feelings were always intense. I can see her spiked yellow hair (sometimes green from swimming in pools with too much chlorine; Tone was a strong swimmer after all), thin ruby-red lips forming into an expression of pure determination, and piercing blue eyes."

Your Legacy

You were never afraid to show your love. You always ended a phone call with your signature "I love ya." And you meant it.

Steve Scheibel says: "There is so much more for me to say about Toni, but most of it would be unfit for public consumption. You see, Toni and I were true friends, we shared everything with each other, and it will always remain that way. Toni, you will be my friend always."

So, we will remember you as a loving mother, sister, grandmother, and loyal friend. How about candid, no nonsense, and brutally honest?

And, in bigger terms, we will remember you as someone who made a tremendous difference in the lives of thousands of people through your HIV work. Tone, we will be talking about you for a long, long time.

And, as for the two of us, Tone, we had so much more to do, much more to see, and a lot more to talk about. We never made that trip to Hawaii, but we will admire the hibiscus for you next time we are there and toast you with a Mai Tai or two.

In closing, Tone: Aloha. AND—we love ya.

Final Thoughts on Toni

Many years later, Toni's daughter, Felice, said that our meeting was meant to be, once again challenging my belief system as a nonbeliever of such issues.

Ordinarily, I would reject this, saying there is no such thing as destiny. On the other hand, after reflecting on those years of knowing Toni and recalling the synergy of our lives together—I can *almost* become a believer.

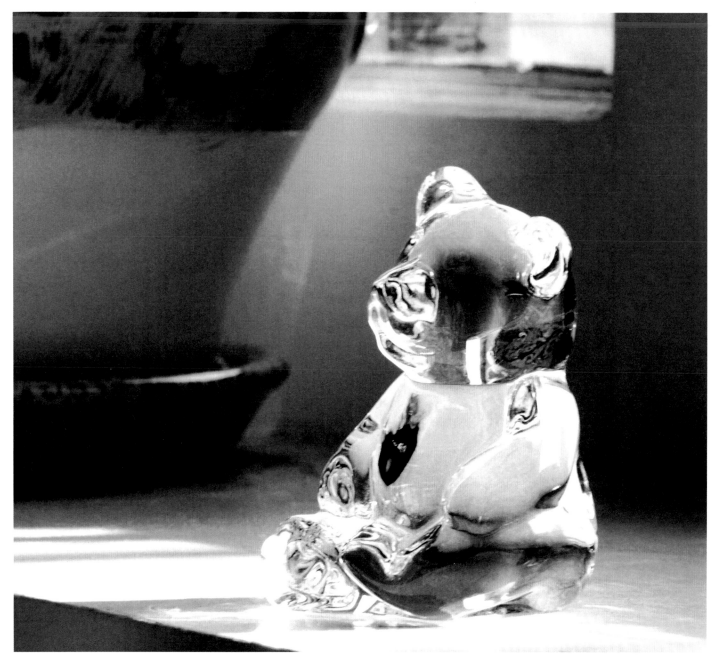

▸ A gift from Fritz and her mother. This glass bear has watched me from the windowsill in my home office since 1990.

19 | A DAUGHTER AND HER MOTHER: "FRITZ" AND RAMONA

We loved having Fritz come to the clinic. She was the kind of
person who seized every opportunity to make things pleasant.

— Sidney Metzger

When I think of Phyllis "Fritz" Hogestyn, the word "guts" comes to mind. Fritz was one of our earliest patients at CHN. As a woman with AIDS, she helped forge a new direction for the movement.

Fritz's mother, Ramona Frank, accompanied Fritz to office visits. Ramona, another charter member of Sid Metzger's Mothers Group, was unique, because it was not her son who was our patient—it was her daughter.

In contrast to our understanding of HIV today, in the early days of AIDS, the information came in fragments—mostly in case reports from the CDC. First, gay men and injection-drug users were identified in 1981. This was the explosive part of the epidemic. After the initial report of the first five cases of what we would later know as

AIDS on June 5, 1981, the CDC reported another 26 cases a few weeks later.

The "Haitian connection," a cluster of cases in Haiti, came a year later in 1982. In December of that same year, a transfusion-associated case

"THERE WERE DAYS WHEN IT WAS US AGAINST EVERYBODY ELSE ... "

was reported in a baby in California. Shortly after that, the CDC reported 22 cases of immune deficiency in babies. Mother-baby transmission had officially arrived as we sat back and tried to make sense of it.

The CDC reported cases of AIDS in female sexual partners of men with AIDS as early as 1983. In Rochester, we saw our first heterosexually transmitted case in a woman two years later, in 1985.

Toni Obermeyer was working at AIDS Rochester when she connected with Fritz. Toni developed a quick interest in women with AIDS.

She, Fritz, and Ramona were a trio to be reckoned with.

Fritz was determined to set the record straight. Never pushy or aggressive, she was the contrary. Calm, thoughtful, and focused, she never let her medical issues get in the way of her role as a spokesperson for people with AIDS—especially women.

Remember, this was the era of stigma that forced people into hiding. Instead of receiving compassion, people were scorned. There were days when it was us against everybody else, although we certainly had people on our side. We realized that part of the job was to provide clear, consistent information to people, and Fritz's campaign did just that.

Steve certainly provided that compassion as Fritz's doctor. Sid Metzger was a part of the effort and forged a bond with both mother and daughter. We were all rowing in the same direction.

When I said that Fritz had guts, I suspect she inherited them from Ramona. Their energy and passion for the cause helped to educate the community by telling the real story. The trio of Fritz, Ramona, and Toni Obermeyer fought to make things better for those who didn't or couldn't have a voice of their own.

Thanks to Steve's stellar care, Fritz had a rebound on AZT and used the time to good advantage. She did countless interviews, television

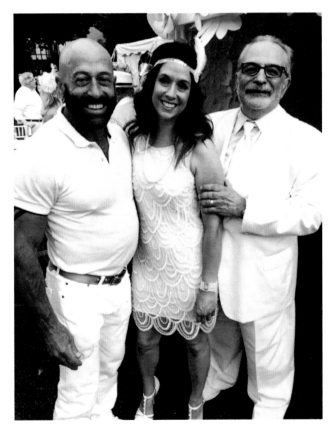

▸ Steve Scheibel, Fritz's daughter Julie Hahn, and Bill Valenti at Trillium Health's 2016 White Party. Julie's family resemblance and smile are remarkable.

appearances, community forums, and talks in churches, often accompanied by Toni Obermeyer. She was also instrumental in forming a support group for women at CHN. I suspect Ramona's love and support for Fritz gave her daughter the horsepower she needed to be the advocate she became, despite her illness.

I have two gifts from Fritz and Ramona. One is a glass bear that has watched over me from the windowsill in my home office since she presented it to me in 1990.

The other is a Santa hat. At Christmas time, 1989, shortly after CHN opened, Fritz and Ramona showed off their sewing talents by presenting us with red, felt Santa hats. The hats had our names in glitter on each: one for Bill and one for Steve. I can still see Fritz and Ramona giggling as I put the hat on my head. I wore it for the rest of the day in the spirit of their thoughtfulness and the bond we all shared.

More recently, Steve and I were reminiscing about Fritz. He reminded me of how he visited her on rounds at the hospital at the end of her life. As they talked, she said, "This is the hardest part—the loneliness at the end." Then, he did something truly remarkable. Fully clothed, including his motorcycle boots, he climbed into bed with her, and they talked. He recalled that the Highland Hospital staff doing her care merely continued their work with the two of them in the bed.

As he related this story all these years later, I shook my head in amazement. Hospital rounds like no other. The bond was that intense and that giving.

A mother of two young children, Fritz died at the age of 40, shortly after Christmas 1990. After she died, our social worker Sid Metzger spoke of her contributions to the effort. "Fritz was courageous, joyful, and proud to be who she was. She fought in a most gracious way to dignify the diagnosis so that people didn't have to hide."

Personally, I remember Fritz as warm, soft-spoken, and always with a smile on her face.

I have known three generations of this family, and it has been a privilege. Fritz's daughter, Julie Hahn, and her husband attend our fundraisers every year and continue to support our efforts.

Julie Hahn, Steve Scheibel, and I were all together at Trillium Health's White Party fundraiser in 2016. Steve had never met Julie. When I introduced them, he said, "Wow. You are as beautiful as your mother. I can still see Fritz." What struck me about the meeting was that after 27 years, Steve remembered Fritz instantly. Quite simply, those bonds are timeless.

WILLIAM M. VALENTI, M.D.

So, what is healing, anyway? It can be anything you want it to be as long as it's loving.

"All the resources that you need to heal are inside you. Your style (and your acceptance of it) is more healing than HIV drugs, organic brown rice or aloe vera.

"These things may heal, but only if they are a part of your design.

—Randy Wickstrom's words on healing. The Personal Medicine workshops funded by his family and friends after his death were based on this philosophy.

20 | A GYMNAST, A DANCER, A HEALER: RANDY WICKSTROM

*Randy's philosophy was that everyone had all the
resources they needed within themselves to heal.*

This was a young man who had been active since he was a child. In fact, he was so active that his mother asked the doctor for help. The prescription: gymnastics. He took to it naturally. And with a lot of hard work throughout his school years, he excelled. After college, gymnastics led to modern dance. Soon he was in New York City enjoying his newly found career. Randy danced; even after he was diagnosed with AIDS, he continued to dance professionally. Sadly, his dance career was cut short by his illness. He came home.

Randy's mother Barbara was another of Sid Metzger's Moms. Another force of nature, my mother would have called Barbara "determined." Steve Scheibel was Randy's doctor. Barbara loved Steve. He walked on water in her eyes.

Despite the best of care and the fight of a lifetime, AIDS took Randy. It was 1990. He was 28.

After Randy died, his family made a generous donation to CHN to establish the Randy Room. The room, in use today, was designed to be a refuge for patients and staff with comfortable furniture and away from the exam rooms. Over

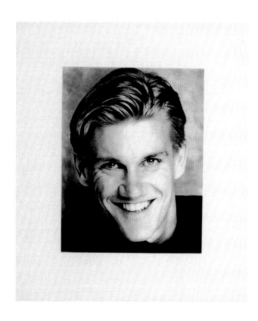

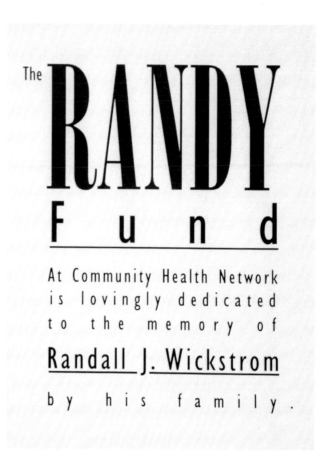

The **RANDY Fund**

At Community Health Network is lovingly dedicated to the memory of **Randall J. Wickstrom** by his family.

the years, thousands of patients and staff have used this room for meetings, support groups, interviews, and other activities.

For a number of years after Randy died, Barbara, Randy's dad Bob, and his sister Wendy

hosted a summer fundraiser at their Brighton home. Dinner under a tent and an auction—a high-spirited get-together to raise money for AIDS.

At one of these parties, as the festivities were winding down, I turned around and saw Barbara and Steve standing and facing each other. She took his face in her hands, looked up at him, closed her eyes, and put her head on his shoulder. They were both reduced to tears.

The Wickstrom family's commitment to honor their son's memory and help others with AIDS was a powerful demonstration of parents' love for their children.

Thanks to the many people attending the Wickstrom's fundraisers, the proceeds were used to fund a workshop series called "Personal Medicine." These workshops were offered to patients at CHN for many years. The purpose of the workshops was to help people find their inner resources and use them to heal.

To quote a headline from the local *Democrat and Chronicle* newspaper article after his death: "A fallen dancer's energy still flows to help others."

The Wickstrom family defines the era of how to turn grief into something enduring and meaningful. I smile a little when I hear our current staff refer to a meeting in "The Randy Room." It's a part of our Trillium Health culture.

Recently, the cast of a touring theater production connected with us through our outreach efforts and came to the office for health screenings. I stopped in the Randy Room where our 20-something patients/actors were waiting to be seen. I told them about Randy and his career and how important he was to our history.

"The past is prologue." Randy lives.

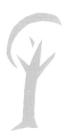

21 | A MATTER OF FAMILY URGENCY

*When they told me that they wanted to have a baby, I scratched
my head and tried to think of a way to talk them out of it.*

It was 1989 when I first met Arthur at Community Health
Network. HIV was in the headlines and in the news every day.
People often went untreated, and when they entered care, they were
very sick. But Arthur found out early and responded well to AZT.
Often, his wife came along to office visits. She was HIV-negative.
We talked at length about how to stay HIV-negative. They became
early, consistent condom users.

Arthur and his wife both did well, and their commitment to one
another was very strong. I was always encouraged to see them together, because HIV had a tendency to split some couples apart. He
had a few rough patches with his health but overall, went to work,
owned a home, and was a good husband.

At one visit in 1998, they surprised me with big news. They wanted to have a baby. I thought to myself, "You've got to be kidding." I thought it was too risky and wanted them to wait.

In 1994, we learned that if a woman was HIV-positive, we could prevent HIV transmission from the mother to the baby by treating the mother with HIV drugs, including AZT. On the

"I MADE IT VERY CLEAR THAT THEY SHOULD CONCEIVE THIS BABY VERY QUICKLY ... "

other hand, making a baby with an HIV-positive father and HIV-negative mother was still uncharted territory in those days. But they were determined. So, my choices once again were to either lead, follow, or get out of the way. I decided to help them find a safe way to have this baby.

I called Steve Scheibel, who was living in San Francisco by then. Together we concocted a regimen for Arthur's wife to keep her HIV-negative during conception and avoid mother-to-baby HIV transmission. Since Arthur's HIV drugs

were working and he had an "undetectable viral load," we gave his wife the same drugs that he was taking plus AZT. Fortunately, these drugs were known to be safe in pregnancy.

Looking back, this was our version of what we now know as pre-exposure HIV prophylaxis (PrEP). In fact, prevention of mother-to-baby transmission of HIV paved the way for our understanding of PrEP as we now know it, although the two ideas were disconnected at the time.

We also developed a plan for her regular HIV testing—every six weeks—during conception and pregnancy. I made it very clear that they should conceive this baby very quickly, because her obstetrician, a former resident of mine, was concerned about the HIV drugs she would be taking. When I consulted with him, he said, "I'll do my part in this, but tell them to speed it up and make that baby." The couple got busy, and they conceived after several months.

Our treatment plan worked. She remained HIV-negative during conception and pregnancy. As a result, their child, a boy, was born HIV-negative, thanks to the good care of our partners at the University of Rochester Medical Center's high-risk obstetrics and gynecology clinic.

We were all thrilled over the birth of this baby. Over the years I got to know the little guy, who frequently came along with his dad for visits, usually with a book in hand to keep him occupied. Arthur would often tell me how well his son was doing in school, so I took some pride in our concerted effort that helped bring this child into the world.

Arthur has been living with HIV for 27 years and is healthy; his wife remains HIV-negative, thanks to condoms and, more recently, the once-a-day preventive pill, Truvada, for PrEP. I always knew in my gut that HIV care would improve over time and that we would eventually be referring to it as a chronic illness. Still, back in 1989, I couldn't have imagined that we would have connected the dots in quite this way. What a journey.

In late 2015, husband and wife came to the clinic for his regular check-up. They were excited to share good news with me—our "little guy" was graduating from high school in 2016. "Best of all," said his proud mother, "he has been accepted at Columbia University on a full scholarship."

I could hardly contain my happiness. The three of us just laughed and hugged. I felt as though my own child had been accepted at Columbia.

As I've thought about this experience, two things come to mind: one, the ability to follow people and their families long-term has been an extraordinary privilege, and two, I love happy endings.

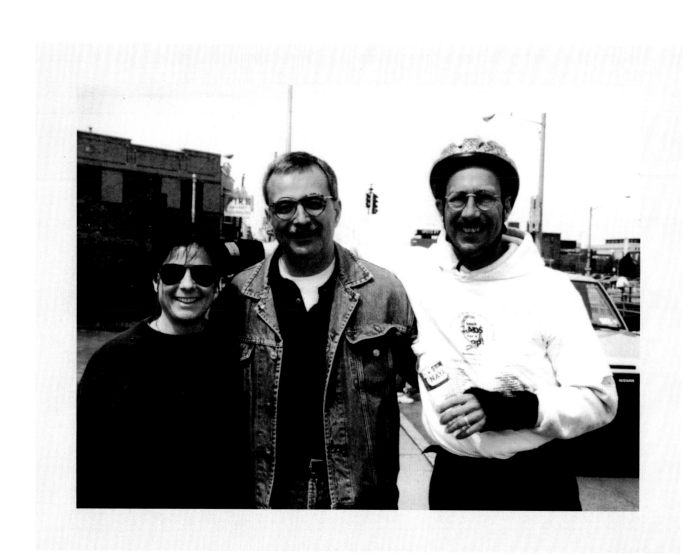

▸ Left to right: Rita Pelusio, Bill Valenti, and Jeffrey Barhite. "Knock AIDS" fundraiser, May 18, 1997. Photo by Garnetta Ely.

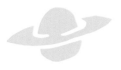

22 | KNOCK AIDS FOR A LOOP: JEFFREY BARHITE, 1950-2014

Jeffrey, we would love to have you here to
help end the epidemic by 2020.

On June 25, 1996, a newspaper article described newly approved HIV drugs. Under the headline "AIDS Drugs Launch Fierce New Fight" is a picture of Jeffrey Barhite and his dog Nikki. The sidebar says that Jeffrey "takes the new drugs but is skeptical about a cure and doesn't think he can ever shake the stress of having HIV."

Jeffrey was one of the early "AIDS warriors." I met him when I first came out as a gay man more than 30 years ago. We were part of the same group of up-and-coming 30-somethings.

Long before he knew his HIV status, he was involved in the AIDS effort. In his first career, he was a teacher. When I met him, he was a hairdresser, his second career. While he cut my hair in his shop on Atlantic Avenue in Rochester, we would talk about the epidemic, our friends, and the need to do more.

When "Helping People with AIDS" was formed in 1986, Jeffrey began to transition his stress into action. He helped HPA become the success that it was for its 17 years of existence.

I understood his passion and knew that he was capable of doing much more for the effort. As the clinic continued to grow, Dan Holland, then Community Health Network executive director, said it was time to hire a full-time development director. We both smiled as he asked me what I thought about hiring Jeffrey.

Jeffrey closed his shop, we hired him, and he launched his third career as the Community Health Network's development director. Around that time, he took up roller-skating. Always in good shape, I'd see him around the neighborhood, gliding by gracefully on skates.

His signature fundraiser, the skate-a-thon "Knock AIDS for a Loop," was a natural for Jeffrey, the skater. Always challenging the status quo, he somehow managed to obtain the necessary permits from both the city and the New York State Department of Transportation to close Rochester's Inner Loop highway on a Sunday morning.

More than 300 in-line skaters, 150 volunteers, and numerous sponsors helped "Knock AIDS" and raise more than $25,000 the first year. Over its four-year life, the event raised almost $200,000.

Thinking back, Jeffrey was an innovator. He found ways to bring his passion for skating to a new level and merged it with his fundraising skills for the AIDS effort. "Knock AIDS" did more than that. It appealed to a demographic that might not have been involved in the AIDS effort otherwise. HPA's audience was Rochester's LGBTQ, allies, and business communities. "Knock AIDS," on

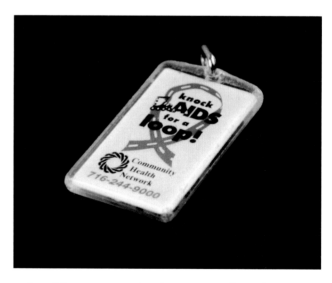

▶ One of the many promotional items created for the fundraiser "Knock AIDS for a Loop."

the other hand, appealed to young people with a passion for skating. This event gave them a skating venue like no other—the Inner Loop. For those efforts, Jeffrey won the Association of Fundraising Professionals Award for Fundraiser of the Year.

After he retired, Jeffrey spent his summers in Ogunquit, Maine, where he continued to make an impact on the lives of people with AIDS. In 2014, Jeffrey died.

A friend and captain of the Ogunquit AIDS Walk's Team Jeffrey remembers him this way: "Team Jeffrey was established in memory of my dear friend and neighbor, Jeffrey Barhite. He lived with AIDS for 25+ years and made each day a great day, always finding something to keep himself occupied. He will never be forgotten by those whose lives he touched."

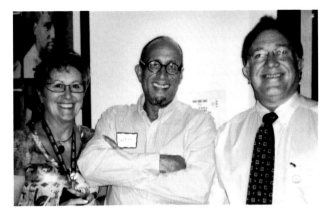

▸ Left to right: Nurse Donna Carlson, Jeffrey Barhite, and Jay Rudman, former president and CEO, Trillium Health, at Community Health Network's 20th anniversary celebration, 2009.

As of 2016, Team Jeffrey was still very much alive and walking in the Southern Maine AIDS Walk—a real tribute to their friend, indeed.

Jeffrey, if you were here today, we would be talking about the end of the epidemic—truly "knocking AIDS for a loop"!

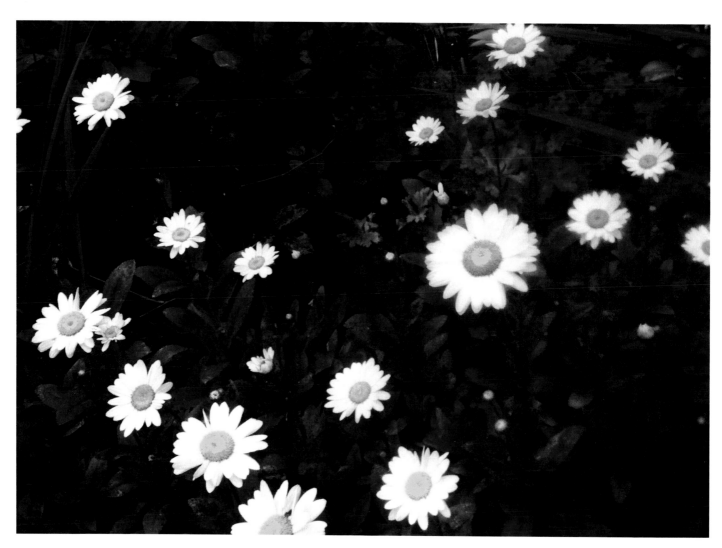

▸ Another era, another garden. These Shasta daisies, a gift of my friend, student, and mentor Joe Anarella still bloom in my garden more than 30 years after he presented me with a clump from his own garden.

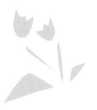

23 | THE FLOWER GARDEN: A METAPHOR FOR LIFE

*She told me she bought flowers for her garden and let
them die without watering or planting them.*

When I first met a new patient in the early 1990s, she had contracted HIV from her first partner in a relationship that lasted a year.
Her brother had died of AIDS two years earlier. She was depressed
and refused to see a counselor. She was sure she would embarrass
her family by dying of the same horrible disease as her brother.

Because of her high level of distress, we used our common interest in gardening as a jumping-off point for discussion during our
visits. One time, she told me that she had bought a lot of annuals for
her garden, never planted or watered them, and let them die. "I don't
care about any of it," she said.

During each visit after that, I'd talk to her about counseling, and
she refused. She wouldn't go for her mammogram either. "I don't
care," she'd say. We continued to discuss the need for counseling.
Actually, I discussed it. She didn't want any part of it.

One of the advantages of seeing my HIV patients so frequently in those days was the opportunity to continue an important discussion over a longer period time. It wasn't always that way for me. When talking to her, I would often recall a transformational moment with a young college student in his 20s when I was a resident on duty in the emergency department.

He came in for one problem, but it appeared to me that his problems went deeper. I asked him if he would like to talk with our "counselor," code word for psychiatrist. He declined.

In the end, there was nothing physically wrong, and I had to release him. He came back by ambulance several weeks later with self-inflicted, irreparable damage to his eyes. It's the only time a patient experience has made me physically ill. I second-guessed myself for years after that. He haunted my dreams.

This experience told me that I needed to change my style. I would never again fail to act on what my gut told me. My duty to patients would forever be a part of my clinical decision-making. I would also push my patients harder to engage in therapy with a qualified mental health professional—and I have. Relentlessly.

After several years of talking about it with this patient, she finally agreed to see a counselor, and something changed. She and the counselor from our in-house mental health program

"SHE TALKED ABOUT THE PIVOTAL TIME WHEN THINGS CHANGED FOR HER AFTER COUNSELING."

clicked. Her mood lightened, and she became more enthusiastic about living. That year and every year since then, she has had a beautiful garden, and her mammograms are up to date.

During a visit in 2016, we talked about then and now. She recalled the early days when she first came into medical care after the shock of learning that she was HIV-positive. She went on, "I remember that day vividly. I can tell you what I was wearing when the counselor told me my test results." She talked about the pivotal time when things changed for her after counseling.

She talked further about how she deals with her HIV today and goes on with her life. Recently, she said, she feels better about herself today than the period before she learned of her HIV status.

Along the way, she started writing children's books. She is extensively published and talks about changing careers and writing full-time. During that visit, she showed me a picture of her garden. It was thriving, with pots and window boxes full of flowers of all kinds, colors, and sizes. More recently, she extended the garden season with a full range of fall flowers.

Good work, my friend! It took some time, but it was worth it.

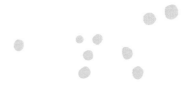

24 | A TALE OF TWO PATIENTS: EVERYTHING OLD IS NEW AGAIN

Out, damned spot!

—William Shakespeare. *Macbeth*

It was 1983. Kaposi's sarcoma was one of the cruelest of the AIDS opportunistic infections. Many patients could hide the raised, purple spots on their skin with clothing—unless those spots were on the face. Adam was one of my patients who moved back to Rochester from New York City. Articulate, soft-spoken, and always beautifully dressed, he had launched his New York career as an investment banker. Now, he had Kaposi's all over his once-handsome face, and he came home to live with his family.

He had been treated previously at two centers in New York City with no improvement. I thought to myself: What now? If they couldn't do anything in New York, I was now on the hot seat.

When he first arrived, he explained how the Kaposi's had started on his neck and spread to his face. Then, he pulled out his driver's license and said, "I used to look like this." The picture on his license in no way resembled the swollen face covered with those purple spots. The only similarity was that the picture showed his blue eyes.

I followed conventional wisdom and sent him to the Cancer Center for another round of chemotherapy—a different regimen than his previous treatments. We waited for improvement.

Fat chance. The chemotherapy wasn't working, and we both knew it. One day, he looked at me with very sad eyes and said, "I know it's not working, doc." Choosing my words carefully, I said what I always said when we were running out of treatment options, "Let's think about this. There's always something we can do." I knew I was backed into a corner, but I needed to give him some hope.

I called Dr. Linda Laubenstein, the Kaposi's expert in New York who first described the Kaposi's/AIDS connection. She said that they had been tracking the herpesvirus link and thought high-dose acyclovir (the herpes drug) treatment made sense, considering our poor understanding of Kaposi's at the time. I noted how she pronounced Kaposi's as "Cop-O-She's" and

not "Ka-Poe-Zee's." I've tried to use the European pronunciation since. Fortunately, the disease has been rare in the modern era, and I haven't needed to utter the Kaposi's word much at all.

Adam was a trouper. During many of his visits, I'd ask him if a few medical students could come into the room so they could see Kaposi's. He was courageous and agreeable. He always said what so many other patients of the era said, "Yes, if it will help someone else."

So, over the course of two years, he endured having people poke at the lesions on his swollen face to see how they lightened in color with pressure. During those sessions, I would explain to the students what we knew about Kaposi's, which wasn't very much.

The Kaposi's lesions in his mouth and on his swollen lips were troubling to him. During one office visit, he told me that he had difficulty swallowing and drooled while eating or drinking; he was embarrassed when it happened in front of his mother. He said that he often ate alone, even though he preferred eating with his family.

I was numbed by the conversation. I went back to my office, thinking about the iron lung machine I'd seen during the polio era. I wondered which was worse? Spending your life in an iron lung when polio paralyzed your breathing or being tortured by Kaposi's and drooling while you eat? And, then eating alone. How much more isolated could he be? On top of that, how about trying to live your fate with grace and dignity?

If we couldn't do anything for his Kaposi's, I thought, maybe we could do something about his swallowing and drooling problems.

My plan initially was gentle radiation therapy to shrink the Kaposi's in his mouth. While driving one day, it occurred to me that speech therapists worked with patients who have swallowing problems. Maybe they could help Adam. Shortly after I made the referral, the speech therapy supervisor stopped by my office to discuss Adam's case. Hesitating, she said, "What would you like us to do? We've never done this with an AIDS patient before." I smiled back at her and said very patiently, "Welcome to my world," and we both laughed. Then I walked her through the dilemma, including the elephant in the living room: can HIV be transmitted by saliva? Transmission by body fluids was still a hot-button issue in those days.

The upshot was that Adam improved with speech therapy teaching him how to swallow. One day during an office visit, he looked at me and smiled. He told me that his swallowing had improved, the drooling had stopped, and he was enjoying eating with his family.

For now, as Adam's disease spread relentlessly on his skin and internally, at least we gave him some relief from drooling in the six months he had left. He died with some dignity restored. After that visit, I sought refuge in my office again and thought that I needed to stop doing AIDS care. It's hopeless, and I can't do this anymore.

Then, I thought of how pleased he was with our compromise. I reminded myself that he was doing the real work here. Adam had to leave his house with his face scarred by those purple lesions. He endured people backing away from him or looking away rather than looking him in the eye. I thought that in light of what he endured, if he could leave his house and if he could elect to eat alone, then I couldn't break the trust he placed in me. I could continue to take care of him and people like him. I felt powerless and hopeful at the same time. I admire his courage to this day. He gave me the boost I needed to continue.

Years later, we would learn that KS was, indeed, caused by a member of the herpesvirus family: human herpesvirus Type 8, to be exact. With the advent of combination HIV therapy, Kaposi's would disappear for the most part.

The Modern Era: The Return of Max

After 1993, I didn't see another new case of KS until 2013 when Max reappeared. He had been lost to care since the mid-1990s. I would see him around town and, *sotto voce,* say to him that I hadn't seen him in the office in some time. He would say that he felt fine and didn't need any follow-up. That is, until he noticed those painful, purple lesions on his feet and couldn't walk.

After a visit to E.D., he was referred back to me. I was shocked when he took off his socks. He had obvious Kaposi's on both swollen feet, in his groin, and, as we learned later, in his lungs. It felt like someone had turned back the clock.

My mind started racing, trying to put the pieces together. After a 20-year absence, Kaposi's was staring back at me one last time. The MASH-unit, war-zone mentality kicked in. As the lesions on his feet blanched when I poked at them, the graph of the modern-era integrase inhibitor class of drugs flashed through my brain. These new drugs result in a huge, sharp drop in HIV in the blood; they work faster and better than any of the older drugs.

This time it would be different with Kaposi's. This would be our big chance to beat down the enemy and get rid of it. I know, the herpes viruses never really leave the body. But this was a chance

> ## " ... WHILE WE HAD ALL KINDS OF HIV DRUGS AVAILABLE, HE HAD NO INSURANCE."

to use modern-era drugs and hope that immune system recovery would carry the day.

Of course, Max had chemotherapy later. I'm not that much of a risk-taker. However, the lopsided dynamic of Max's current situation was that while we had all kinds of HIV drugs available, he had no insurance. That was never a problem before. It shouldn't be a problem in 2013, I thought. Trillium Health's millennial reinforcements would come to the rescue.

I pulled our clinical pharmacist into the room. I explained that we had a matter of urgency here. New Kaposi's, no insurance, and we needed modern drugs today. "I'll take care of it," was her quick response. She put the regimen together, and our pharmacy dispensed the drugs. The lack of insurance would be solved later. It was a relief to have a pharmacy on hand as the contemporary version of the bottom drawer of the nurse's desk of Adam's era. Max started treatment with an integrase drug that day.

Could starting drugs that day have waited? Sure, but wait for what? More KS lesions to sprout up all over Max? Spread to his lips and mouth like Adam? What were we waiting for? For him to drool while eating? The team was there, and we could start treatment that day, and we did. After 30 years, Trillium's mantra was still to provide "barrier-free care," in the manner of its Community Health Network legacy.

While Max was under the watchful eye of our treatment counselor who made sure he took his medicine as directed, a group of us would converge on the exam room to monitor those miserable spots on his feet and scrotum. In contrast to Adam's case, this Kaposi's was disappearing before our eyes. His chest X-ray started to clear. This time, the KS experience was almost joyful.

During those monitoring visits, I saw Shakespeare's Lady Macbeth in my mind—holding her hand in the air, guilt-ridden over the murders she left in her wake, imagining blood on her hands, and shrieking "Out, damned spot!" Over the course of Max's treatment, I acted out that scene from *Macbeth* to anyone who cared to watch. Those "damned spots" disappeared in six months.

More importantly, I thought of the sharp contrast between these two patients over 20 years. People like my long-ago patient, Adam, made the real contributions to the effort and were the real heroes. Adam died, but he laid the foundation for the success with Max.

Adam, Max, and my skilled colleagues all did the heavy lifting. Once again, I was merely the catalyst.

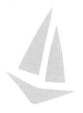

25 | A TALE OF TWO DOCTORS: YOUR SECRET'S SAFE WITH ME

I finally had an idea of what it would be like if I were in a situation similar to my patients.

Some of what I've learned over the past 35 years is to anticipate what might lie ahead based on the decisions I make today. Anticipation, I've also learned, is an imperfect science. Sometimes, it helps; other times it doesn't. Still, some advance planning is better than none at all.

Before the HIV test was licensed in April 1985, the test was done at a state approved lab, anonymously and by number; no names were used. I kept testing materials in the trunk of my car, ready to test anyone on a moment's notice. I was a familiar face at the lab in those days.

Weekly, I dropped off tubes of blood at the lab for HIV testing. Each tube was carefully numbered and logged in by the lab chief. She and I kept identical log books with names and numbers. We kept our book in a locked box in a locked drawer in the clinic.

After the HIV test was approved for patient use in 1985 and HIV drugs were available, a group of friends and I decided that we would all get HIV-tested together. It seemed like a good idea when we cooked it up. Toni Obermeyer was in the group; she said she would probably be positive, considering her past history of injection drug use and sex work.

We met at Steve's house and made it a social event. We decided that, considering the sensitive nature of this, we would do the testing anonymously, by number. After dinner, we drew each other's blood and logged our names and numbers into the book.

A week later, the lab's medical director called. One of the tests was positive. The confirmatory test was also positive, making it a done deal. "Are you sure?" I asked, hope against hope. He said we could repeat the test just to make sure.

I checked the logbook. It wasn't Toni Obermeyer. It was Steve Scheibel.

I sat there, numb—and thought about how to deliver the news. I was rehearsing in my head how to do it. An HIV diagnosis is a life-changing event. The implications are different for each patient and their families. The goal is to manage the negative impact on the patient. Delivering this news was never easy.

My stomach was in knots all day, a lifelong feeling in times of stress. In her gentle way, my mother called them "butterflies in your stomach."

" ... WE WERE BOTH IN A HEAP ON THE FLOOR CRYING WITH MY ARMS AROUND HIS SHOULDERS ... "

If that was the case, then a colony of very large butterflies had set up shop in my gut. In reality the feelings were panic, fear of death, anger, isolation, loneliness, why Steve?

At the end of the day, I went to Steve's house unannounced. I made a lame excuse about stopping by when he met me at the door.

The next thing I remember after telling him the test results was that we were both in a heap on the floor crying with my arms around his shoulders while he sobbed on my shirt.

I told him that we would repeat the test and that the results would be back in a week—a lifetime for someone on edge. In the meantime, we would use the time to plan his treatment.

The hard decision was how to treat him to avoid the word getting out. We decided to create a chart using a pseudonym. He became a back-door patient, and his office visits blended with his time in clinic. Fortunately, he was healthy, did well on the antiretroviral drugs of the era, and required only T-cell monitoring.

Doing his care under a pseudonym was risky for all of us. We did what was needed to shield him. In this case, the downside of being more public would most likely have interrupted or ended his career. We did not want him to have to deal with what we tried to avoid in the rest of our patients—including stigma.

Would we create a pseudonym again? We never did. It was a different era then. Desperate times demanded desperate measures.

Steve, of course, engineered his own treatment, so it was a unique experience and has remained so. Over the years, he has kept himself healthy with advances in HIV treatment. More than that, he has been on a journey in a career where he has made significant contributions to advance the science that has benefited many other patients as well.

My Turn: A Calculated Risk

1990 did not start out well. Shortly after Community Health Network opened, I had a needlestick while drawing blood from a patient. I took AZT for a month. It made me sick, but I got through it, even though I felt like I was in a fog for a month.

Shortly after I finished the AZT, I was diagnosed with prostate cancer. A relatively minor problem led to prostate biopsies that led to the diagnosis of low-grade prostate cancer.

I remember when my urologist called me on the phone to deliver the news. I took the call in Steve's lab. The butterflies returned as I listened to him describe the biopsy results. He told me that he recommended surgery. I thought, "I can't die now. I'm too young." I had the same feelings that I had when I learned of Steve's positive test results—panic, fear of death, anger, isolation, loneliness, why me?

I was still defining my sexuality. Not now. I was still doing HIV tests on my potential sex partners. Foreplay consisted of mutual HIV testing. In fact, I had testing kits in my refrigerator at home, just in case. Cancer was impossible for me to fathom. I was crushed, immobile.

I felt like the floor had dropped out from under me, as though I was in a free fall. Dazed, I landed in Carol Williams's office and delivered the news. I remember her reaction. The mothering Carol put her arms around me and consoled me. The thoughtful Carol wanted to think about this in her "problem-solving mode."

She advised me to talk to Steve and to get a second opinion. The only option recommended at the time was surgery, and I didn't want that. I went to Steve and he pondered the situation further. We discussed a multitude of options and plans for treatment. In the meantime, I had two "second opinions" from other prostate cancer experts. The answers were both the same—surgery.

Ultimately, Steve and I decided on a regimen of alfa-interferon and isotretinoin (Accutane), both powerful immune system stimulators. We had considerable experience with interferon but none with isotretinoin, a vitamin A family member used for severe acne treatment at the time.

When I finally presented this idea to my urologist, he scratched his head in amazement. After a long discussion, he agreed to a compromise if we combined it with his monitoring plan. We would do periodic prostate scans and biopsies and watch the prostate-specific antigen (PSA) test. The "watch-and-wait" treatment plan worked for me. Watch and wait is an important current-day option for prostate cancer. At the time, it was risky, and I knew it. On the other hand, I had faith in Steve's avant garde approach and decided to go for it.

I did the treatment for a year. The standard interferon injections of the era, in contrast to today's modified version, had major side effects. I had fatigue and headaches much of the time. The treatment was difficult, yet vaguely familiar. I now had some inkling of what my patients were experiencing with a serious, potentially life-threatening illness with treatment that made them sick.

I never had surgery, and I have not had a recurrence of prostate cancer. Over the years, my urologist has chuckled over the risk we took that worked.

Similar to many of my patients, I opted for non-disclosure. Steve, Carol Williams, Sid Metzger, and my medical school roommate Bruce Hinrichs were the only ones in the know. It wasn't until many years later that I told anyone in my family.

I was, in fact, like some patients. I was being monitored, looking for alternatives, taking a risk, albeit a calculated risk. I thought of how this would interrupt my life. What saved the day was what we had pioneered—thinking ahead, careful monitoring, and an exit plan. The exit plan in my case was that I would have surgery if there were any signs of cancer.

Together, Steve and I survived our health crises. The work, difficult as it was, proved beneficial. It was a necessary distraction and probably better than trying to make sense of the conflict over our physician roles that required us to be strong for our patients when we both felt so personally weak and vulnerable. Add this to the relentlessness of the work and the fact that we both had "domestic" issues that we were juggling at the same time.

Life circumstances affect the way we handle news like this. Steve eventually told his parents, even though they weren't accepting of his being gay. Their reactions were mixed, with little response from his father. His mother, perhaps prophetically, spoke of his strong immune system.

As for me, I went into denial. I was the AIDS doctor, and I was frightened to death at the thought of surgery. I didn't want to draw attention to myself or be labeled weak or vulnerable. And, after witnessing AIDS stigma, I didn't want to be seen as a cancer patient. What I failed to accept or understand was the fact that I *was* a cancer patient.

Steve and I were there for each other during the best of times and the worst of times—and always will be. Words are inadequate to express our gratitude for the colleagueship and friendship we share.

I remain in awe of Scheibel's mind, not only for what he continues to do for the AIDS effort but what he did for me. I have no doubt that he could well be a major player as we move to end the HIV epidemic.

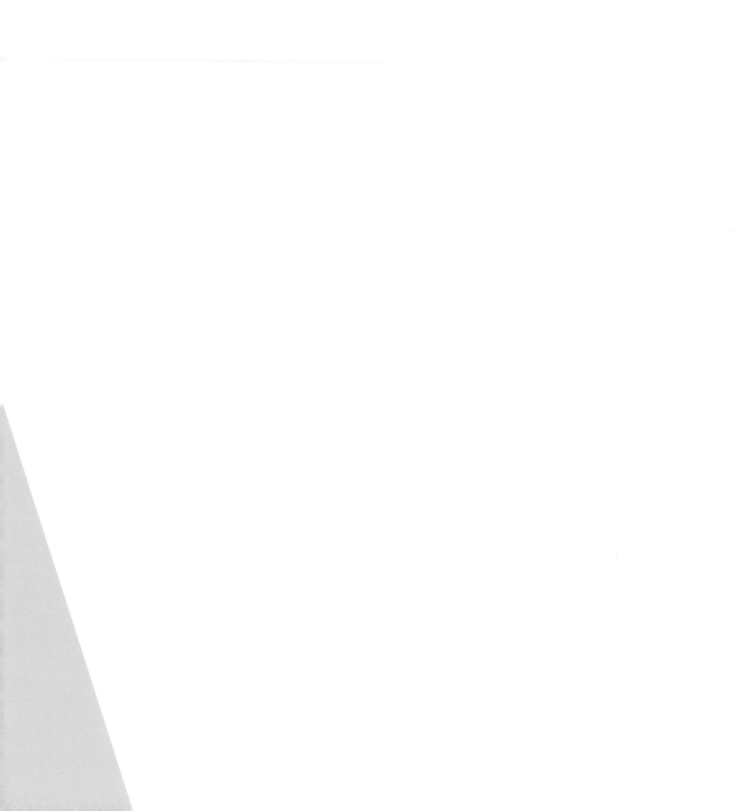

A LOCAL CHRONOLOGY

We had no idea when we read those first reports of
AIDS how the world or our lives would change.

1981

▸ First cases of AIDS reported by the U.S.
Centers for Disease Control by Michael
Gottlieb, M.D. Dr. Gottlieb was a graduate
of the University of Rochester School of
Medicine and Dentistry and was an internal
medicine resident at the University of
Rochester Medical Center.

1982

▸ Screening clinic set up at University Health
Service to screen men who have sex with men
for AIDS by Thomas Rush, M.D., and nurse
practitioner Sue Cowell.

1983

▸ Care of AIDS patients moved to St. Mary's
Hospital under the direction of Raymond
Mayewski, M.D.

▸ AIDS Rochester established by a grassroots
group of local people to respond to the AIDS
crisis.

▸ Rochester Area Task Force on AIDS (RATFA)
established by the New York State Health
Department. Bill Valenti, M.D., and Jackie
Nudd, the first executive director of AIDS
Rochester, are founding co-chairs.

1985

▸ HIV care moved back to Strong Memorial Hospital's infectious diseases clinic.

▸ The first HIV antibody test is approved for patient use.

1986

▸ AIDS Clinical Trials Unit established at University of Rochester Medical Center.

▸ 101 new cases of AIDS reported in Rochester.

1987

▸ AIDS Vaccine Evaluation Unit established at University of Rochester Medical Center.

▸ HIV: AZT approved by the FDA as the first HIV drug.

▸ Strong Memorial Hospital designated an AIDS Center Hospital by the New York State Health Department as part of New York State's initiative to ensure that HIV care was available throughout the state.

1988

▸ The University of Rochester infectious diseases unit leads the initial trial of didanosine (ddI), the second HIV drug licensed by the FDA.

▸ AIDS Training Project established at the University of Rochester Medical Center with a grant from the National Institute of Mental Health.

▸ Rochester Area Task Force on AIDS and the Finger Lakes Health Systems Agency publish their report on AIDS in the Finger Lakes Region. The report projects that the number of AIDS cases in the region will double over the next 10 years.

▸ AIDS Resource Library established at Monroe Community College as a community resource, funded by Monroe County government.

▸ Rochester Roman Catholic Bishop, Matthew Clark releases his pastoral letter. "A Pastoral Instruction on the AIDS Crisis," to the community.

▸ December 1 is designated World AIDS Day by the World Health Organization. An ecumenical religious service was held at Third Presbyterian Church. Jackie Nudd, executive director of AIDS Rochester, and Bill Valenti, M.D., spoke at the service. Volunteers distributed red AIDS ribbons to the attendees.

1989

▸ 64 new cases of AIDS reported in Rochester.

▸ AIDS Memorial Quilt is displayed in Rochester at Monroe Community College in May.

▸ Community Health Network opens in July for patients while the clinic is still under construction.

1990

▸ 81 new cases of AIDS reported in Rochester.

▸ Steven Scheibel, M.D., leads Community Health Network's trial of Remune, a novel vaccine for treatment of people living with HIV, developed by Dr. Jonas Salk, who developed the polio vaccine in the 1950s. Remune is still under review by the U.S., Food and Drug Administration.

▸ Michael Keefer, M.D., becomes director of the Strong Memorial Hospital HIV Clinic and starts his signature community outreach activities in Rochester and the Finger Lakes region.

1991

▸ Amy Portmore, M.D., becomes director of Strong Memorial Hospital's HIV Clinic; Michael Keefer, M.D., becomes director of AIDS Vaccine Evaluation Unit, now the HIV Vaccine Trials Network.

1992

▸ AIDS Memorial Quilt displayed in Rochester.

Adapted from a timeline created by Michael Keefer, M.D.

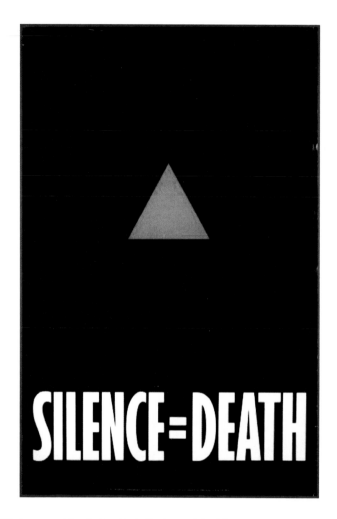

▸ In 1987, six gay activists in New York City formed the Silence = Death Project and began plastering posters around the city featuring a pink triangle on a black background stating simply SILENCE = DEATH. In its manifesto, the Silence = Death Project drew parallels between the Nazi period and the AIDS crisis, declaring that "silence about the oppression and annihilation of gay people, then and now, must be broken as a matter of our survival." The six men who created the project later joined the protest group ACT UP and offered the logo to the group, with which it remains closely identified.

EPILOGUE | ENDING THE EPIDEMIC BY 2020
ETE 2020: FINISHING THE JOB

I never imagined that today we would be talking about ending the epidemic.

This is 2017. A high-stakes game to end the HIV epidemic by 2020 was unthinkable during the early era. If EtE 2020 succeeds, this will be the most significant public health initiative of this century. Even if we come close to the goal, EtE 2020 is a game changer that will have been worth the effort.

In the 1980s, we were trying to get ahead of the epidemic in a different way. We had a lot of sick patients, no drugs to treat them, and no technology to monitor them. We were also hampered by AIDS hysteria, a crying need for public education, fear of contagion, stigma, and the sluggish response of the political establishment.

Today, EtE 2020 is the end game, a rallying point that has reignited the discussion of HIV. The idea of ending the epidemic is possible because of the groundwork laid by the original treatment teams everywhere. Our patients' and their families' tremendous courage and sacrifices also helped move the needle to this point.

Locally, the Rochester community's response to the AIDS epidemic was focused and generous at every level. "Just tell me what I can do" carried the day. People created fundraisers, attended fundraisers, opened their homes and gardens for events, wrote checks, connected us to their contacts, offered advice, and volunteered their time.

Again, the response in Rochester was a small piece of the movement that was replicated hundreds of thousands of times in communities worldwide.

Our local Gay Alliance of the Genesee Valley (GAGV) provided regular AIDS updates in its *Empty Closet* newspaper from the beginning. Editor Susan Jordan has been a consistent presence on the "AIDS beat" since 1989. In fact, GAGV began Rochester's Pride Parade in 1989 in response to AIDS and was organized by Rochester ACT UP leaders Paul Scheib and the late Martin Hiraga. In May of that same year, when the NAMES Project Memorial Quilt came to Rochester, GAGV held a quilt workshop in advance and made 30 Rochester quilt pieces to display.

New York State's more than 30 years of sound HIV public health policy has proven to be a wise investment that allowed us to translate innovations in technology, drug development, and research into the care of patients. The early efforts of people like Dr. Nick Rango, the first AIDS Institute director, followed by my long-time AIDS Institute collaborators, Dr. Bruce Agins, Lyn Stevens, Dan O'Connell, Colleen Flanigan, Ira Feldman, and Karen Hagos, all of whom passionately carried out Nick's vision, set us on the path to EtE 2020.

After almost 30 years, I continue to admire the dedication of my colleagues on the AIDS Institute's Quality of Care and Medical Criteria Committees.

Since 2014, my fellow members of New York State's Ending the Epidemic Task Force have worked tirelessly to create and implement the Blueprint to end the epidemic. It is an honor to be a part of this effort. Now, Johanne Morne, the newly appointed AIDS Institute director, has the responsibility to lead us through to 2020.

The Medical Society of the State of New York (MSSNY) has been a critical force in the movement. While I have been chair of MSSNY's Infectious Diseases Committee since 1990, Patricia Clancy, vice-president for Public Health and Education, has kept me focused, on schedule, and relevant.

AIDS advocates deserve a major share of the credit for bringing us to this point and for opening my eyes to the reality that the movement would have more horsepower as a medical/community partnership. In fact, EtE 2020 was the brainchild of two New York City advocates,

Charles King and Mark Harrington. Fortuitously, these two visionaries conceived the end of the epidemic during a brief incarceration after a protest in Washington D.C. People like Michael Callen, who woke me up to the movement, laid the groundwork for King and Harrington.

The EtE 2020 initiative won't cure HIV. That will come later, but I suspect Dr. Steve Scheibel will be a part of finding that cure. I once told him, jokingly, that if I had a billion dollars I'd give it to him to find a cure. His calm and serious response was, "I could do it for less!"

EtE 2020's concerted effort puts the goal within our reach—to bring new infections to "sub-epidemic" levels to fewer than 750 new infections statewide by the end of 2020. The three key elements of EtE 2020 are quite fundamental: (1) more HIV testing to link HIV-positive people to care, (2) retaining those people in care to achieve an undetectable viral load that prevents transmission to others, and (3) offering the one-pill-a-day pre-exposure prevention (PrEP) to HIV-negative people at risk. We've been doing it this way since the beginning of the epidemic by pulling together. The difference is that we now have the tools, experience, and passion to make it happen.

If we don't make it to fewer than 750 new HIV cases in New York State by 2020, we will come very close. The stakes are too high not to. Now, my millennial colleagues will step up to the plate. They continue to inspire me, and they will continue the journey long after 2020 to an AIDS-free generation.

They will be the people who finally finish the job and deliver us to a world without AIDS.

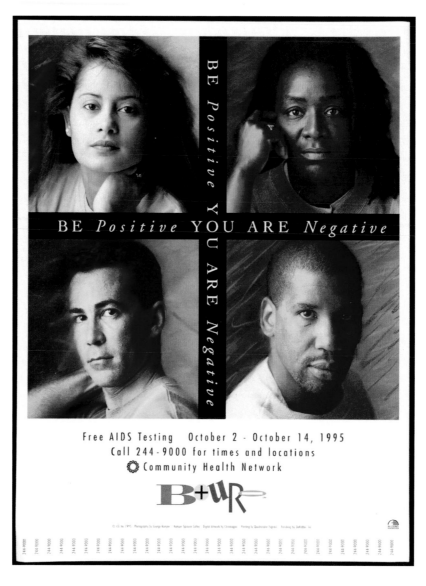

▸ "Be Positive You Are Negative." Community Health Network's community HIV testing campaign ran for several years starting in 1995. Jointly sponsored by the Rochester Primary Care Network, the initiative helped us spread the testing message to people of color. Examples of this campaign are in the Trillium Health/CHN Archives and in the Atwater Collection of AIDS Education Posters, University of Rochester Rare Books and Special Collections.

ACKNOWLEDGMENTS

Whatever I've accomplished was done with the assistance of thousands of people, some of whom are recognized below. The list is endless. I know I will miss some names, so I hope people will contact me and gently remind me.

Patients and Families

Those who agreed to participate in this project by telling their stories.

James Wolk, my partner, my muse, for your endless patience with "Just another email, and I'll be ready to go."

My brother Jim Valenti, Esq., and his wife Susan, who joined the movement and put AIDS house parties on the map after I came out to them at Tom Wahl, Jr.'s house.

My brother Richard Valenti, his wife Mary Ann, my sister, Elizabeth Muscato, her and husband Bob for their endless support, love, and encouragement.

Linda Wolk who kept up the pressure and Dr. Jeffrey Cane for the use of the penthouse to film this book's promotional video.

Karen von Sauers, my high school history teacher and family friend, who taught me that losing was also an opportunity to do other things that mattered.

My extended family whose endless words of encouragement and love erased any self-doubt I might have had over my career path.

Editorial Team

Virginia (Gini) Keck, my friend and editor, who also walked the walk as a patient's mother.

Martha "Martie" Last, Ed.D., my cousin, for her wisdom on the art of storytelling.

Brandon Capwell, Carrie Tschetter, Phil DeCicca and Elaine Lennox, my colleagues at Archer Communications, who guided me through this effort from the beginning.

Matt Wittmeyer, videographer and photographer, whose visual artistry brought this project to life.

Linda Coleman, proofreader, for her attention to detail.

Mary Guhin for her bloodhound detective work that tracked people down for permission to appear in this book.

Advisors

Richard Tubiolo, Esq., Anna Lynch, Esq., Paul Nunes, Esq, and Bob Greenebaum, CPA, for their wisdom that allowed the story to be told.

Members of the Boards of Directors of Community Health Network and AIDS Rochester whose leadership challenged the status quo that saved thousands of lives.

Irwin "Irv" Metzger, Sid Metzger's husband, who became a friend and trusted advisor.

Marvin Hoffman, M.D., former Blue Cross Blue Shield of Rochester vice-president of medical affairs, who taught me how health insurance works.

Richard Gangemi, M.D., my first chief resident and a role model as a clinician/administrator— a class-act in both.

Mentors, University of Rochester Medical Center

R. Gordon Douglas, Jr., M.D., my first chief of infectious diseases, and Clifford B. Reifler, M.D., director of the University Health Service, both superb physician administrators, who took a chance on my passion and limited experience and helped shape my career.

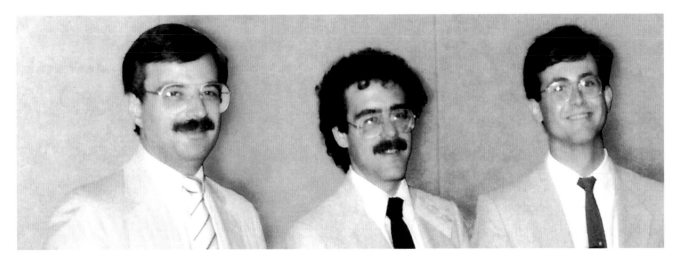

▶ Left to right: Bill Valenti, Bruce Agins, Joe Anarella at an infection control meeting, Washington, D.C., 1984. Anarella presented our paper on health care workers' understanding of AIDS.

Robert F. Betts, M.D., infectious diseases mentor, who helped me translate the data into patient care.

William Morgan, Jr., M.D., who coached me for my first AIDS grand rounds presentation. "If you are prepared, you will know more about the topic than anybody in the room."

Margaret D. Sovie, Ph.D., R.N., former dean of nursing practice, who taught me how to leverage responsibility into advocacy.

My Students Who Became My Mentors

Joseph P. (Joe) Anarella, MPH, who allowed me to pay it forward and take a chance on someone with passion and limited experience.

Bruce Agins, M.D., AIDS Institute medical director, who taught me that the quality of HIV care should be a global movement.

Tadd S. Lazarus, M.D., whom I met as an inquisitive resident. As an HIV physician and, later, as a leader in the biotechnology industry, he advanced my understanding of diagnostic technologies in fighting the fight.

Clinical Team

My fellow providers over the years at all levels who broke new ground regularly and kept the vision alive.

My Tuesday evening clinic colleagues for their commitment, good humor, and endless patience with meeting my needs.

Those who thought that Community Health Network wouldn't make it. We listened to you and addressed those doubts to ensure that we succeeded.

My medical colleagues who have consulted on our patients from the beginning. If anyone was fearful of AIDS, they never showed it in the excellent care they delivered in those early years.

My many nurse colleagues who followed in the footsteps of Carol Williams: Carol Plank, R.N., Jane Reid, R.N., and nurse practitioners Mary Angerame and Craig Sellers.

My social work, care management, and other colleagues who addressed the social determinants of health and overcame thousands of barriers to keep patients engaged in care.

My infection prevention colleagues who helped refine my thinking on matters of contagion.

Arlene Van Halle, the Community Health Network "adult amidst the chaos."

Friends, Organizers, and Volunteers

Our AIDS Walk participants and volunteers, who walked thousands of miles for the cause.

Our AIDS Red Ribbon Ride bike riders and volunteers for their endurance, stamina, and camaraderie.

The Greater Rochester Eastern Area Tournament (GREAT) and the Rochester Historical Bowling Society, whose bowling fundraiser for CHN, starting in 1990, raised hundreds of thousands of dollars over more than 25 years. Carol Williams opened the first tournament and bowled a strike. We were on our way.

My loyal friends and donors to the effort who became community organizers and mobilized, spread the word, networked, wrote checks, created and attended fundraisers, referred patients, and encouraged me from the earliest days of the epidemic.

Hugh "Kelly" Gaspar, David "Dash" Hamblin, and Dr. Albert Jones who curated the beginnings of Community Health Network's collection of joyful, hopeful art donated by community artists.

Joanna Hodgman, volunteer extraordinaire, for her dedication to the cause and for keeping us organized in those early years.

My fellow members of Trillium Health's executive leadership team and our chief, Andrea DeMeo, for embracing EtE 2020.

The staff and board of directors of Trillium Health who continue to advance us toward 2020.

Media Partners

Over the years, television, radio, and print media reporters, editors, and writers have taken the time to allow me to tell the story. Thank you, all.

Pharma Partners

My colleagues from the pharmaceutical industry who joined the fight in the earliest days and have continued the march to 2020.

PERMISSIONS AND REGISTERED TRADEMARKS

The author gratefully acknowledges the following permissions:

Permissions

Cover Art: *Dance* by Michael Chiazza (modified), 1989. Used with permission.

xvi   Photograph of a protest. Courtesy of Lisa Brozek. Used with permission.

xviii   Dining for Dollars XIV poster, artist unknown. Helping People with AIDS, Inc. Collection of Trillium Health/Community Health Network, Rochester, New York. Used with permission.

xxv   *Break Thru* by William N. Copley. Copyright © 2017 by Estate of William N. Copley/Copley LLC/Artists Rights Society (ARS), New York, New York. Used with permission.

xxvi   Photograph of John Altieri, Sue Cowell, and Bill Valenti. Courtesy of John Altieri. Used with permission.

6   Photograph of Drs. Susan E. Cohn and Bill Valenti. Copyright © University of Rochester, Rochester, New York. Used with permission.

10   Photograph of Dr. John Wendell Washburn, Jr. Collection of the John Washburn Library, Trillium Health/Community Health Network, Rochester, New York. Used with permission.

15   News clip, "Task force on AIDS is formed in Monroe." Copyright © *Democrat and Chronicle*, Ancestry.com Operations Inc. Reprinted with permission.

22   News clip, "You can't lie to them." Copyright © *Democrat and Chronicle*, Ancestry.com Operations Inc. Reprinted with permission.

26   Photograph of Minnie Mouse decal. Copyright © The Walt Disney Company.

34   Photograph of Dr. Steve Scheibel and Dr. John Washburn. Collection of the John Washburn Library, Trillium Health/Community Health Network, Rochester, New York. Used with permission.

48   *Mother and Child.* Copyright © Kathleen Hanney, Rochester, New York. Used with permission.

68   Photograph of Opening Day, Community Health Network, December 1989. Collection of Trillium Health/Community Health Network, Rochester, New York. Used with permission.

80   Photograph of Sidney Wilson Metzger. Copyright © Tantalo Photography, Rochester, New York. Used with permission.

88   Photograph of Bishop Matthew Clark. Copyright © Greg Francis, photographer, and the *Catholic Courier*, Rochester, New York. Used with permission.

108   *The Angel Book.* Copyright © Karen Goldman/Simon and Schuster.

160   Silence=Death poster. Copyright © Manuscripts and Archives Division, The New York Public Library, New York, New York. Used with permission.

164   Be Positive You Are Negative poster. Copyright © Community Health Network, Rochester, New York. Used with permission.

167   Photograph of Bill Valenti, Bruce Agins, Joe Anarella. Copyright © Association for Professionals in Infection Control and Epidemiology (APIC), Arlington, Virginia. Used with permission.

        An Event in 3 Acts. Design Industry Foundation Fighting AIDS (DIFFA), New York, New York.

        The NAMES Project AIDS Memorial Quilt. The NAMES Project Foundation, Atlanta, Georgia.

Registered Trademarks

AZT (azidothymidine; Retrovir®). ViiV Healthcare UK Limited, Brentford, Middlesex, United Kingdom.

ddI (didanosine; Videx®). Bristol-Myers Squibb, New York, New York.

March of Dimes®. March of Dimes Foundation, White Plains, New York.

Apple® II computer. Apple, Inc., Cupertino, California.

Remune®. Immune Response BioPharma, Inc., Atlantic City, New Jersey.